A
PHYSICIAN'S
Apology

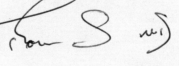

Alison —
Wishing you Tons of
Smiles and Health!
Hugs & Love Galore.

Thomas Schneider, M.D.

from S m)

INDIGORIVER
PUBLISHING

A

PHYSICIAN'S

Apology

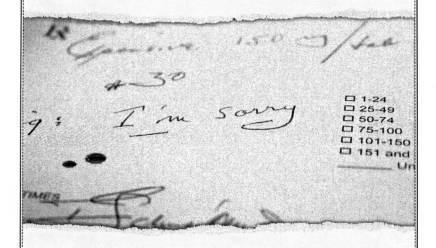

Are WE making you sick?

Thomas Schneider, M.D.

A Physician's Apology: Are WE making you sick?
Copyright © 2013 by Thomas Schneider

Editors: Adam Tillinghast, Matthew Jordan, Donna Melillo
Cover Design: Jason Kauffmann / Firelight Interactive / firelightinteractive.com
Interior Design: Rick Soldin / book-comp.com
Illustrations: Julie Clark O'Brien

Indigo River Publishing
3 West Garden Street Ste. 352
Pensacola, FL 32502
www.indigoriverpublishing.com

Ordering Information:
Quantity sales: Special discounts are available on quantity purchases by corporations, associations, and others. For details, contact the publisher at the address above.

Orders by U.S. trade bookstores and wholesalers: Please contact the publisher at the address above.

Printed in the United States of America

Library of Congress Control Number: 2013936317
ISBN 978-0-9891263-0-4

First Edition

With Indigo River Publishing, you can always expect great books,
strong voices, and meaningful messages.
Most importantly, you'll always find . . . words worth reading.

Dedicated to:
Mark, Kristy, Ellie, Robert, Missy, and ...
Truth.

"Everything in moderation—even moderation."
—Oscar Wilde

Contents

CHAPTER 1

A Physician's Apology

APOLOGY: *A written or spoken expression of regret, remorse, or sorrow for having insulted . . . , injured, or wronged another.*[1]

*I*know what you're thinking—another book on wellness or health?! You don't think you can handle it—I'm not sure that even *I* can handle it. But I do think that there is a place for a book about truth in all the literature about "wellness" that inundates us all.

As a physician who deals in healthful living and preventive medicine, I'll give you my best definition of wellness. I actually have to give credit to my wife's 96-year-old aunt. She recently fell and fractured her hip (which is essentially a death sentence for anyone over 80 years old). I got on the phone with her and said, "How are you feeling?" Her frail answer was simple: "Better than yesterday."

That may very well be the best definition of "wellness" that I've ever heard because that's what it's all about, isn't it? ***Feeling better today than yesterday***—now, that might be as simple as having a different outlook about your spouse or giving him/her a compliment

---

[1]Dictionary.com

today. Or perhaps it means having a little less pain in your day, taking an extra step, engaging in a new sport, or even just smiling more. The list, of course, can go on and on—it just depends on your life and how enthusiastic and innovative you are.

I have added a tad more to her definition. To me, wellness also includes having vitality and energy every day with or without disease. Yes, that's right—with or without it. You may be ill; you may already have diabetes or heart disease; and you may already have pain. It doesn't matter. This book is about the truth on how to become better every day. It's going to take baby steps to get better, but together we can do it.

It is *not* the goal of this book to create a new you. No, you're not going to wake up and suddenly find yourself to be a Brad Pitt or Nicole Kidman look-a-like. But by taking these baby steps, I can assure you that you will be a better you.

This book is about the *truth*, and here are the two primary principles of that pure truth that you must understand:

Principle #1: It's going to take small, everyday changes to just maintain who we are today, both medically and physiologically. This is a really important concept to grasp from the start. You may say that staying the same is a bit frightening, and it might be. But the point here is to not get worse—to stop the bleeding. That's the first step toward wellness. Once we've reached a certain level, we can begin to take baby steps for improvement.

Principle #2: If it ain't simple, it's not sustainable. It has to work for you every day in every way, and you must see signs of improvement. Otherwise, you're just not going to continue. You have to take it day by day and step by step. For instance, I'm ready to go to Krispy Kreme right now; but my game plan this morning seems to be working, so I'll hold off at least until tomorrow.

There is one key to learning about how to get to your "better": finding the *truth* about the information that doesn't have our health and well-being in mind. The truth is the most difficult information to decipher in today's world. It's even harder to find than Bin Laden was. So here's my first apology: Truth is extremely hard to find in medicine and science, and I'm sorry. The words medicine and science conjure up truth. They even suggest sincerity and good wishes, but where was the truth when it came to tobacco (causes cancer), low-fat foods (loaded with fructose and transfats), and Premarin (pregnant mare urine, which also causes cancer)?

Let's face it: this is a commercial world, and the bottom line is always the buck. Where do we find the truth? It's hidden way under that green paper stuff—money!

I sat back one evening and flipped through the 860 channels on my television. At least half of them were infomercials on how to get ripped abs, get a larger penis, have better orgasms, or lose 100 pounds in just 3 months. Do any of those sound totally absurd to you? Come on—seriously? The truth is that those claims are absurd, and you don't need me to tell you that; it's just common sense. But somehow, in the midst of all of this commercialism, common sense and truth are often buried.

Throughout this book, I'm going to tell you a number of medical and scientific facts that are different from what many have always been told. Why believe me? The truth is you shouldn't. Believe the *truth*. Feel free to check out the resources at the end of the text and look up the facts that I state. Check them all out. All of this information is available to you on the Internet and through a host of other sources; it's just been obscured by a sea of commercials and creative marketing.

I will list the most important resources but not an endless number of them. Why? Because I know you probably won't go to them. If you're like me and the rest of the world, you don't have time. You also won't find pages and pages of recipes made with exotic herbs and spices that I don't have the time to find.

Again, so why believe me? I certainly don't have all the answers nor am I the bastion of truth. But I do have fervor for the truth. In fact, I'm about to tell you a true story; but first, I want to give you an honorary M.D. degree. No long hours or on-call nights—just POOF! You're a doctor. Now before you get too excited, I'm also going to give you your first patient.

What do you do when a man in his late 60s comes to your office for an evaluation and help? He's married, and he was a former fighter pilot in Vietnam. He was shot down and landed in Agent Orange, which is known to cause all sorts of metabolic and physiologic abnormalities. Somehow, he made it back from the war and went to medical school. He is also a physician, but he certainly didn't take very good care of himself during all those long hours. He smoked; he drank; and sleep was simply not a concept that he snuggled up next to.

In 1994, your patient developed a number of issues. So yes, he started a "wellness program" for himself. He was running triathlons and came down in weight from 294 lbs to 180 lbs. Good for him! He was no longer smoking or drinking, but he was still working long, long hours. During one of his triathlons, he noticed some shoulder pain and was subsequently diagnosed with coronary artery disease. This progressed to bypass surgery and then, subsequently, five coronary stents. He also developed diabetes during this time. After being given medications that destroyed his kidney function, he was put on dialysis. His kidney function did come back; however, he was given more medication to alleviate some of the aches and joint pain. This medication perforated his intestine, and he ended up spending 3 months in an Intensive Care Unit for the repair of a perforated bowel. He was also diagnosed with cancer, which was surgically removed.

About this time, your patient wanted to name himself Mr. Lucky. His medical disasters continued and included such things as high cholesterol, high triglycerides, gout, hypertension, impotence, full-blown diabetes (requiring insulin), and a bunch of other fun stuff. He now arrives at *your* office, doctor, and wants to know if what he's been doing for himself to stay alive has been worthwhile. Are you ready to meet your patient?

Well, that patient is me! Yes, that's exactly what happened to me over the last 18 years. And no, my "wellness program" of triathlons and overworking was *not* worthwhile. A commitment to a healthy living lifestyle plan cannot be bottled like a pill—even if that pill is a triathlon, a super-supplement, or a can-do attitude (in the face of a can't-do body).

Fortunately, I met a number of very bright and progressive physicians, and we developed a program to evaluate patients holistically. Not much of this medical path had been published yet; it was a question of digging and finding the right answers and then applying them to me. We are going to discuss many of the concepts of my treatment here. No, these are not paradigms that most physicians are going to describe to you or even know about. Nonetheless, they are indeed the *truth*.

There is one last important point I'd like to make before we get started. This book is meant for learning the truths of healthy living and how they apply to *you*. I am often called "doctor" by my patients. Do you know what the word "doctor" means? No? Neither do most *physicians*. When I teach at medical schools, I ask the students or the newly graduated doctors to tell me what their title means. I often get the response that it means "healer" or "curer." Some are so brazen to say "guardian of a patient's health." Wouldn't it be nice if these were true? Sorry, they're not. "Doctor" comes from the Latin word *"docere,"* which means "to teach." That's right; a doctor's mission is to *teach* patients. But we doctors haven't done a very good job of that, and I'm sorry. Part of it has to do with economics, time, fatigue, and just a lack of knowledge; but the fact remains that we very seldom teach.

So here's my advice: If you visit your physician for any reason and receive a prescription, ask about the prescription and its complications. Review the meeting you had with your physician and see if you were taught anything about yourself or your health. If you haven't, find another doctor. I'm sorry.

CHAPTER 2

The Rules

"Find the truth and live it!"

—Me

So you may ask—why an apology? Well, my purpose is to set the medical record straight and put some sanity into our world of healthcare. Even if healthcare providers, the media, pharmaceutical companies, or even your good ol' Aunt Louise have the best of intentions, the information we are given is often just plain wrong (or, at best, is unsupported by scientific evidence). Lord knows I am struggling with the system, so my guess is that you're looking for a lifeboat as well.

I know that this may sound a tad arrogant on my part, and I'm sorry, but many physicians consider the word "M.D." after their name to signify "minor deity." I can assure you that my "M.D."—as you now know from my medical history—stands for "major disasters." But I think I have learned from them.

My day has just a few goals: *Enjoy. Give. Teach the Truth.*

No, I'm not a monk—I'm far from it. I'm just adamant about finding out what is simple and what works. Then, I take it one step further—I don't stick to just that sole solution. I try to modify and challenge my "truths" every day. Every health and wellness book usually says at this point something like, "Be sure to notify your physician and get a checkup prior to beginning any medical program." Well, this isn't a medical program; this is a lifestyle change, and it's a chance for you to be the director of it. As you continue reading, there are some basics for you to know and to be confident about. Here are some of them:

The Basics

1. *You know your own body and its limits.* Be confident in that knowledge. I know you're not going to do anything goofy like suddenly decide to run a marathon if right now you have trouble getting from the sofa chair to the bathroom. You're bright; you're intelligent; and you read. Right now, do the sane, simple things that will help your body. Most of all, as you begin this new learning experience, realize that it's not a prison sentence. This is a gift you are giving to yourself—after all, it's about time, right?

2. *Educate yourself.* Hello—this is the 21st Century, and we have the Internet. There is a host of educational formats available that you can use to teach yourself about how to prevent diseases as well as treat the current diseases you may have. Unbiased and factual medical information will equip you to better interact with your physician when customizing your personalized health plan. Here's my caveat: Look for the pure informational sites like the National Institute of Health (nih.gov), medscape.com, or pubmed.com. These sites are designed solely to educate the consumer and have no bottom-line interest in selling you a particular pharmaceutical product. Refer to the appendix for a list of the unbiased sites. (I'm not sure you'll use these any more than if I gave you recipes, but

these will be solid sources of information for you if you choose to learn more.)

3. *Don't diagnose and treat yourself.* I know that's kind of a given, but I have to mention it because it comes up every day. Patient after patient will say to me, "Aunt Martha took ginger root, and her gout is gone!" Well, good for your aunt. That has nothing to do with science or validity. Her gout probably just died out. Do, however, become your own prevention expert. By that, I mean *prevent* yourself from disease every single day through your choices. Now, I don't want you to walk around frightened about the germs on every shopping cart as you walk through the grocery store, but I do want you to realize that there are some sane things you can do (including frequent hand washing) that will keep most common and difficult diseases away. We'll discuss more about that in a tad.

4. *Work with your doctor toward disease prevention.* I'm saying this because it makes obvious sense to me, but perhaps not to your doctor. I've mentioned it already, but I'll say it again: if you've seen your physician and haven't learned something new about yourself (meaning you haven't been taught anything), find another doctor. You're not going to the doctor to get another TV-advertised purple pill for heartburn; you're going there to find out why you have heartburn in the first place. Once you find out *why*, then we can work on the parameters that will keep it from coming back. I don't know about you, but it sounds pretty simple to me, and yet it's seldom done. For every illness, find the 25th letter of the alphabet—Y.

5. *Don't treat others!* This is another straight-up, self-explanatory statement, but I'm always running into patients who have been treated by Aunt Martha. They come in with concoctions, diets, or over-the-counter medication treatments for literally everything— including diseases they don't have and will probably never get.

If a friend comes to you with a medical problem, bite your lip regardless of what you just heard on NPR or Oprah. Send him to the best preventive physician or best-caring physician that can deal with his problem. If a friend comes to you with a headache, please don't offer him an aspirin. Why does he have a headache? Is it a subdural hematoma? (How's that for a biggie for you to look up?) Is he allergic to aspirin? Does he have an ulcer? A host of problems can arise from just the simplest of over-the-counter medications, and you do not want to be the one responsible. You do want the best for him, however, so give him the name of the best physician you can find.

6. *Trust your common sense.* All right, this one's a real toughie. Not only is truth hard to find, but right behind it is common sense. I'm not sure common sense even exists anywhere anymore. (Just take a flight on our airways in the United States, and you'll understand. Good grief! Does anyone think the measures we use would stop a terrorist? Please forgive me; I sometimes rant.)

Common sense doesn't exist in the medical field; everyone just wants a miracle pill. That's the way we've been raised, and that's the way the American economy wants it. We believe there has to be a pill to solve every problem, and we certainly don't need to worry about why a particular disease, pain, or complaint happened. Wrong! I'm sorry—but if anything sounds too good to be true ... Okay, I'm not even going to finish that statement because you already know it. I mean—seriously—do you really think you're going to get six-pack abs in six weeks? Do you really think you'll be a better lover after taking a little blue pill? And here's the best one—is there any pill that's going to give you a longer life?

Now please don't take me to be a curmudgeon. There are plenty of wonderful supplements, activity programs (Pilates, yoga, resistance training, etc.), and cognitive programs that will enhance your lifestyle. It's essential to find what is going to work for you, and it's important to not beat yourself up. I don't care how much you love the treadmill; after half an hour, you're just an overworked hamster. In a nutshell, it's all about common sense, a commitment to change, and the truth.

The Approach

We've just covered the basics—good for us! Now what do we do? We need to follow what I call the symphony approach. A symphony is not made up of notes nor is it made up of a single violin. A symphony requires a coordinated, orchestrated set of instruments, notes, human beings, and knowledge. The same is true with any medical condition you may have.

Let's look at nasal congestion. That seems simple, right? Most people would take a nasal spray or an antihistamine. I'm not saying that either is bad, but the truth is that nasal spray can easily become addictive. Antihistamine can make you impotent, gain weight, be drowsy, experience dry mouth, or cause a host of other issues. If your congestion is short-term, maybe lasting only three or so days, then sure, give either of them a whirl. But the basic question is *why*? *Why* do you have a runny nose? Is it because of a local allergen, food intake, chemical exposure, another medication, bed mites, dust, diet sodas, depression, stress, or something else?

Now don't become too fearful; most of the time nasal congestion is just nasal congestion, and simple measures can be taken. But the point is that regardless of the symptom or disease, always ask yourself (and hopefully your doctor will also ask) the 25th letter of the alphabet—Y. The symphony approach means you first define *why* you have the runny nose and then eliminate the cause agents.

A doctor may suggest that his or her patient lose some weight. Often, the answer from this physician is to exercise, and doesn't that make sense? No! (By the way, if this advice is coming from a doctor whose only obvious experience with a treadmill is as a clothes hanger, common sense might encourage you to look else where for your treatment.) We'll go into far more detail about this all in the weight section of this book, but in most cases, a treadmill is no more than a pill. That's right—a pill. You must first ask the question and determine why weight is a problem for you. Is it from stress? Is it from anxiety? Is it endocrine dysfunction? The reason has to be defined so the solution can be determined based on the cause. Sure, a treadmill may minimally—yes, minimally—help. (Personally, I prefer a nice, gentle walk in the neighborhood.) The point is that it takes a symphony to lose weight in a healthy way. This approach is absolutely the only way that a medical path can be successful. There are multiple issues that have to be addressed to overcome obesity, and they can't all be conquered with a treadmill—I'm sorry. Don't believe me? Look around—even in gyms! This is such an important point that I'm going to make sure we are all on the same wavelength by the end of the book.

Now if you've got your big boy or big girl pants on, let's get started.

CHAPTER 3

What's Healthy?

*"A dying person once told me that her
sweetest breath would be her last."*—Me

*"Wellness and health means having energy
and vitality with or without a disease.
Cognitive positivity is of paramount importance."*
—Me

In other words, "Think good thoughts."
(I think I can; I think I can.)

I hope that you're not counting on me to tell you what's healthy.
I'm supposed to, I guess, because I'm the doctor. The truth is
that "healthy" changes every day, and "healthy" is specifically defined
by ... drum roll ... you! That's right—*you* decide what's healthy for
you. You set the goal, and you set it daily. The emphasis is a *commitment* to a daily exercise of change. Maybe it's an index card for you.
It is for me. I write down exactly what I'm going to do (or going to
try to do) on an index card. Sometimes, it's taking 4,000 steps that
day. Other times, it's soup for lunch instead of pasta. Maybe it's
to not forget my fiber or even just to compliment my wife. It really
doesn't matter what actions or what the goals are—I get to set them.
It's critically important that you do the same. You may not need an

index card, but you need to write a goal every day. It's just like the annual dental appointment—unless it's written down or someone else reminds us, it just ain't gonna happen. If it's important to you and you want to help yourself commit, write it down.

So how about I give you a couple of "pearls," or mnemonic devices, that we can all remember—even on the day that your daughter comes home with a purple mohawk.

First, you've got to make your goal SANE:

(S) **Simple and done daily.**

(A) **Active.** The goal must require some sort of activity on your part. (Naps are fine, but they just don't count here; sorry.)

(N) **Notice change.** It is important for you to be able to monitor change—whether it's weight, sleep pattern, mood, or something else. I use an index card or notebook for this, and it works for me. For you, it may be a passing notice; but be sure to notice. You're down a half a pound? Unbelievable! You remembered to give your spouse a compliment? Phenomenal!

(E) **Enjoyable.** Whatever you are doing in terms of an activity program, an appetite program, or a cognitive program, you've got to like it. *If it's not enjoyable, it's not sustainable!*

SANE is essential for success. I really don't want to beat you up about this concept of change, but it is critical for your overall lifestyle decisions. You must first choose to be healthy. That's right; it's a choice. It is a choice to make a change as well. I think Yogi Berra has everything in the world attributed to him from a philosophical standpoint, and I suppose he would have summed up wellness with this phrase: "If you don't make a change in your direction, you are going to end up where you are heading." Yeah, that pretty much puts life in a nutshell, Yogi, and I couldn't agree more. Unfortunately, change is never easy; you have to *choose* to make a change.

Second, I use the mnemonic "ACE" when it comes to change because it describes what is required from all of us:

(A) **Awareness.** Prior to a making change, are we even aware that there is a need for it? When I was a fighter pilot, there was no need to change. As a doctor, I had no need to change. The titles I held conferred health immunity on me (or so I thought). Remember my health history? I guess we all need to be open to change. So what exactly needs to happen? That is all definable under the A—awareness. We need to be aware of our needs and aware of the necessary steps to accomplish the change.

(C) **Commitment.** This is self-evident, but it requires a specific, daily commitment. It can't be, for example, a decision to simply improve your attitude—that's too vague. There must be specific steps outlined, and you must go over them every single morning as the day begins.

(E) **Excuses, be gone!** If you have committed to 2,500 steps of walking, then do it. It's just that simple. You may say, "But my knee hurts today." Okay, let's find out *why* your knee hurts. Maybe you don't walk 2,500 steps that day, but those steps are going to have to turn into rowing, walking, or resistance training. You get the picture? Excuses, be gone. Sorry!

I am not going to baby you with a lot of the usual mamby-pamby like "It's time for you to change" or "Today is the first day of the rest of your life." You are way beyond those clichés. You have decided to change, and all I can say is good for you! And I really mean that. It's not great for me; it truly is great for you. My questions to you are how are you going to change, and what does that change mean?

Well, I can only tell you what works for me. First of all, my changes have been tiny steps. That's right; I said tiny, not little. So if I walked 2,500 steps yesterday, my goal today is 2,505 steps—or maybe 2,525 steps if I am feeling overly energetic. The point is that it's just a *small* change. If I ate twelve Hershey's kisses yesterday, my goal is to try to cut down to four today. Oops, I overshot. Okay, six was great for today.

I know you get the point that change is really a marathon—a slow-paced marathon. It's not a sprint. If you have not lifted weights before, don't plan on doing high weights and high-numbered reps. If you do, you'll ache like a son-of-a-gun tomorrow, and you won't pick up weights again.

This is a game plan that I use. All that is required is a short, daily checklist. Again, I use index cards; but for you techies, use whatever you'd like—iPhone, iPad, or whatever your wiring is for the day. Here's the real point: we need a daily, written guideline that anchors us to solid ground—particularly for the days that we're tired, grumpy, or frankly don't even care. Now it would be nice to have one card that you keep on your dresser as a baseline. Remember that we are talking about change, and the only way to define that is to have a base. So on an initial index card, write down your general energy level on a scale of 1 to 10. Also, list your weight, your BMI (body mass index), your percentage of body fat, and your waist-to-hip ratio. Now there is a number of other criteria that you can use, but those are fairly standard in terms of defining avoidance of disease. For example, if your waist is greater than 35 for a woman or 40 for a man, your risk for diabetes and coronary artery disease quadruples.

The BMI is based on a formula that puts your weight over your height (lots of graphs/apps do this for you so you don't have to work out the math). It really is a matter of correct body fat enhancing your prospects of healthy living and disease prevention. Since body fat is difficult to track unless you have an impedance weight scale, the BMI can still be a good guide. Keeping your BMI under 25 is a major

General Energy Level	4
Weight	227
BMI	29
% Body Fat (optional)	28%
Waist/Hip	1.05

Goal for tomorrow:

Grams of carbs: 60

Activity: Row 20 min
Walk 20 min
10 min

Breathing Meditation

Compliment my spouse/partner

Read something different for myself
(for ex: Wikipedia Sisyphus)

Re-do card 1 once a week

goal for disease prevention. You can recheck this weekly, but keep the card in view. You are not going to be able to run away from the cards because they will be staring at you every day to complete and encourage your change.

One little point to remember about your BMI is that they can, in some cases, be notoriously inaccurate; but they do act as a guide otherwise. If you have a large muscle mass, your BMI may indicate that you are overweight or obese since it does not incorporate percentage of body fat. (For example, a muscular, athletic NFL linebacker could be very fit at 6'1" and 240 lbs., but a simple BMI measurement would indicate obesity. In this case, the BMI would be a false indicator because the percentage of body fat would be very low in relation to muscle mass.)

Determining your percentage of body fat can be done in a variety of ways. A simple impedance scale for home use will do a fairly accurate job. Total body immersion in a water tank is extremely accurate but impractical. Using calipers on various body-skin folds is cumbersome and very user unfriendly. A dexa scan (yes, the same one that's used for bone density/osteoporosis evaluations) is extremely accurate and costs under $100. Lastly, an MRI is very accurate but obviously quite expensive. For men, a percentage of body fat less than 22 is ideal. For women, it's less than 28.

To measure your waist-to-hip ratio, use a flexible tape measure while standing with your abdomen relaxed. Measure your waist with the tape at the level of your belly button. Hip circumference should be measured around the widest portion of the buttocks with the tape parallel to the floor. The waist-to-hip ratio should be less than 0.9 for men and 0.8 for women. Do you need some simpler math to work with? Try this: your waist in inches should be one-half your height in inches. For example, a man who is 6 feet tall (72 inches) should have a waist no larger than 36 inches. If your waist measurement is more than one-half your height, you are at a higher risk for coronary artery disease, diabetes, a stroke, and more.

Now, on that second index card (see next page for example), write your goal for the next day—and it can be one or several goals such as decreasing caloric intake, increasing steps, increasing exercise time, increasing meditation time, giving compliments to your family, spending time with the children, or—wow—taking time for yourself to just enjoy life, to name a few.

These index cards may seem trivial, but they truly become of paramount importance. If you are trying to lose weight, for example, it's important to simply take a card and write down everything—food, drink, candy—that passes through your lips. Yep, you heard me right—everything. This will give you a great baseline for where your weight is coming from. We will talk about a number of ways to sanely reduce fat later.

Okay, so now have you really decided to make a change? Really? Okay, let's make it definitive. What are the changes that you want to see, and are they realistic? For example, say you are currently 240 pounds, but you want to be 160? Not in the next 3 months! Probably not in a year, but yes, it can happen with 2 to 3 years of commitment. How do I know? Simple math—1 pound lost every 2 weeks is ideal. Did I go from 294 lbs. to 180 lbs. in 4 months? Nope—it took me 4 years!

Here are a few final points on change:

1. I mentioned earlier that you'll find a phrase in every text regarding healthcare that reads something like this: "Do not undergo any medical changes or treatments without the supervision of your physician. Have a physical examination and checkup prior to instituting any physical activity." Now, honestly, is there anybody alive today that needs that kind of advice? I mean, it's sort of like when you fly on an airline, and the flight attendant comes down and shows you how to buckle your seatbelt. I think there should be a law that says if you don't know how to put a seatbelt on, you shouldn't be allowed to fly in an airplane. I am not going to treat

General Energy Level

4

Weight

227

BMI

29

% Body Fat (optional)

28%

Waist/Hip

Goal for tomorrow:

Grams of carbs:

60

Activity:

Row 20 min
Walk 20 min

Breathing Meditation

10 min

compliment my spouse/partner

Read something different for myself
    (for ex: wikipedia sisyphus)

Re-do card 1 once a week

you like a child because I know you have common sense, and this is nothing more than common sense.

2. Hey! It's the new millennium. Still smoking? Just stop—need I say more? You don't need to hear all of the negatives about smoking—they're just facts of life that you have to accept, like the fact that green means go and red means stop. There are no more excuses for smoking. If you still smoke, try to find out why you hate yourself so much. Why do you want to die? You wouldn't take a sip of snake venom every day. Well, you would be better off with the snake venom than you are with smoking. That includes all kinds of tobacco use.

3. What about alcohol? Well, the latest research shows that one drink per night may have beneficial effects. The operative word there is *may*. Alcohol is an inflaming agent; and as such, it shows very little evidence for any type of benefit to the human body. If it is enjoyable and one drink per night helps to relieve stressors, then fine. What? It's actually two or three? Why not just use lighter fluid? You don't *want* to increase inflammatory stress in the body, but alcohol and tobacco do exactly that.

4. This is a good place to mention the "silent" inflammation process in the body. We'll talk about inflammation a little bit later, but it has to do with stress. Yes, you may have emotional stress that is caused by your children's low grades, your spouse's depression, your job, or any one of a hundred other emotional factors that affect your day-to-day life. But this silent inflammation can also be tied into a systemic stress response leading to such things as alcohol and tobacco abuse. It can also be brought on by taking in inflammatory products such as trans-fatty acids and high carbohydrate foods. I call it "silent stress" because we often do not notice it. Nonetheless, it continues for years and then ultimately shows its ugly head by instigating diabetes, hypertension, or coronary

artery disease. This silent inflammation is the entire core of what this book is dealing with. We want to create a SANE symphony where, over the course of our lives, we manage to dampen that silent inflammation.

5. Are you sedentary? Are you overweight? Are you having trouble sleeping? Is stress a major player in your lifestyle? If any or all of those apply to you, you are just not healthy. I am sorry. So let's do it—let's do something about changing those aspects of your life.

CHAPTER 4

Good News, Bad News

"Over the long term, you are more likely to fool yourself than others."—Nassim Nicholas Taleb

So here we are in the 21st century, and there really is some good news. Today, more than ever, just about any disease can be diagnosed, and most can be treated. Sometimes, you have to machete through a lot of bushes to get to the campsite though. You have to get past tired physicians, improper diagnostic testing, and a lack of personalized care—but proper diagnosis and treatment can be found. Another piece of good news is that we have a wealth of valuable information available to us right at our fingertips thanks to that modern marvel called the Internet. For unbiased medical facts, you can go to websites like nih.gov, medscape.com, or pubmed.com. The Internet is also home to journals, blogs, Facebook, and a host of other arenas that provide information and a sense of community with others who may have your illness or problem. The good news is that this entitles and empowers us all to manage our own healthcare.

More than ever, we truly are responsible for the care that we are going to accept and the care that we stay away from.

We hear a lot about genes determining our fate today, so here is more good news: genes make up just 20% of our medical profile. Just because your dad may have had prostate cancer does not mean that you are going to get it. If Aunt Matilda had diabetes, you have a great likelihood of living a happy life and avoiding it. Heredity doesn't necessarily predict a future heart attack. It doesn't necessarily mean that we are *going* to have those diseases, but it does remind us of particular paths that we may be more susceptible to. Say you have a family history of colon cancer; that is an excellent signpost that says colon screening, within reason, is a good idea for you. Please notice that I said "within reason." As I mentioned, reason and sanity are very hard to find today. Let's look at colon cancer for a moment. If you have a family history of colon cancer, a colonoscopy at age 40 or 45 or maybe 50 is certainly appropriate. If the test is negative, there is absolutely no reason for you to have a colonoscopy every six months; every 5 to 10 years will suffice. Sanity, reason, and always remembering that *you* are responsible for your health are key. *You* are entitled to the evidence and facts.

So let's stick with the good news. There are some easy things you can do every day to decrease your weight if your baseline indicators like waist circumference and body fat percentage are high. Now I am not going to preach to you the way you hear it in every radio ad, newspaper, magazine, textbook, or television show. When I say decrease weight, I mean precisely that. I don't mean losing muscle; I mean losing actual fatty tissue. It won't happen by eating card-board, and it won't happen by starving yourself—I promise you that. There are many factors that are essential for your success and overall health; some are briefly mentioned below. We will get into how in just a little bit.

I've got more good news: your activity program doesn't have to be miserable. In fact, it *should* be fun. It needs to be set and established and defined, but it can involve literally any activity or combination of activities. It can be golfing, gardening, rowing, jogging, walking— you get the picture. Just get some activity every day. My weight loss patients do simple body exercises such as 50 squats in the morning, 50 pushes against a wall at lunch, and 50 biceps curls and shoulder presses with soup cans every night. Is that too much? No problem. Do what you can. It doesn't have to be much; it just has to be *something*.

Along with consistent exercise, it's really important to investigate a low-carbohydrate diet, a low-glycemic index diet, and/or a Mediterranean diet. The good news is that the right foods can actually be delicious, satisfying, and enjoyable. There is a slew of books and articles about nutrition, and some of the best are listed in the back of this book. We will go into a little more detail about nutrition when we get to the section on—yep, you guessed it—diets! I promise you this section won't really be about diets; it will be about you, your goals, and sane eating.

I mentioned sleep a couple of chapters ago, and it is critically important that you understand why. (Yes, I'm going to tell you that it's okay, even essential, to rest your weary body—that's good news, right?) If you are trying to lose weight like most Americans today and you are not getting a restful 7 to 8 hours of sleep, it's just not going to happen. Why not? Without the proper type of sleep and the proper ratio of REM to non-REM sleep (REM stands for rapid eye movement), your body will not be able to produce the hormones necessary for sugar control in the morning. You will get out of bed, and your cortisol level will be astronomical. You will crave sugar. Your insulin level will climb, and that will engender more cravings for brownies and pistachio ice cream (two of my favorites!). So sleep is critically important. Sleep apnea, defined as a number of episodes during your sleep in which you are not oxygenating enough and your body tissues are not receiving enough oxygen and energy, is an epidemic in the United States. We will talk more about sleep hygiene and how important it is; but for right now, go to bed! Make the room dark and take the T.V. out—or at least turn it off. Think about using melatonin (1–5mg) at bedtime for a restful sleep. Another great choice is magnesium (500mg) at bedtime. Magnesium has the added advantage of muscle relaxation (including the heart muscle) and enhancing sugar absorption into muscle—a real perk for diabetics. What happens if you take too much? You'll get mild diarrhea. Magnesium is a winner.

Here's more good news: you *can* be happy. Although we haven't discussed it yet, happiness is one of the requirements for good health. On the surface, "happiness" is a simple word, but it's such a difficult concept to get a hold of that I am going to devote an entire section later on to what it really means and how to get there. I promise. For now, keep this in mind: decreasing stress is one of the great ways to be happy, and I can tell you that it unquestionably comes from the mind. It is not going to come from your children's grades or your spouse's successes. It has to come from you, and it has to come from within.

The next piece of good news is that there really is a heavy promotion in homes, workplaces, and schools for trying to establish a SANE appetite and activity program. Now don't get me wrong—there is no question that healthy nutrition will enhance your metabolism and defense mechanisms; but broccoli and asparagus are not going to *cure* cancer. They may help to *prevent* it, but they sure as heck are not going to *cure* it. The health statements that are strewn throughout our literature and magazines aren't going to cure it either. If you have cancer, get it cut out, radiate it, or use the current best treatment protocol: chemotherapy. The key is this: let's work on trying to not get it in the first place. Okay? We do that by utilizing an activity program like yoga or resistance training and an appetite program that allows you to enjoy food, but just as not as much of it as you might like. The whole purpose of these programs is to initiate a wellness virus in America today. It needs to start in every single business. If you are the owner of a business, this is a great opportunity for you to start it for your employees. If you are in a corporation, you can start it from the ground up, building a cultural change for wellness.

Many large corporations are already involved in this change—and some in an outstandingly wonderful way. Change can be as simple as a green cafeteria. It doesn't mean that there can't be fries and burgers, but there may be a green shelf for green, healthy items. And if you are eating off that green tray, perhaps someone in your company will walk around and give you a gift certificate for Starbucks or a movie pass. It has to be a cultural change. Use the stairs, not the elevator. Oh, look! Halfway up the stairs, there is an apple or some peanuts waiting for you. Well, you get the picture. This type of workplace is ideal to having a healthy living environment because we spend so much of our time at work. The goal of this type of program is to bring this lifestyle home. Bring it home to your spouse and to your children. As you'll see when we talk about an activity program, my daughter, my wife, and I workout together. Now we can't always do it; but for the most part, we shoot for a family activity program and a family workout session. It comes down to the phrase: "The family who pumps together stays together."

Now it's time for a little bad news, folks. (I'm sorry.) The medical system as it exists today is still broken in spite of the best efforts and intentions of so many. For example, you are given a treatment for an upset stomach, and your physician prescribes an antacid. You go home, and your symptoms seem to abate. What haven't we done? You know. We haven't found the why. *Why* do you have an upset stomach? Are stressors in life adding to it? Are you developing a pernicious anemia? There is literally a host of questions to be evaluated. (Are your current medications causing it? Do you use alcohol or tobacco?) Taking an antacid relieves your symptoms, but the process of inflammation continues. And it continues until your next episode—which may show up as a kidney stone. Why a kidney stone, you might ask? Because the calcium you were taking in your antacid has now built up calcium oxalate kidney stones. I could go on and on. My point is that if you have been raised in our system today, we treat for acute illness. It involves a treatment and then a blank period when all seems well until the next medical disaster, and you are then treated until the next medical disaster. Much like the peace time/war time analogy: the best thing to do in peace time is to work for the avoidance of the next war. Get the picture? The doctor treats an acute illness, and then you do nothing. The doctor treats a medical disaster, and then you do nothing. You go back to the doctor for the next acute illness, and then you do nothing—it is those "do nothing" blanks in between that I am going to be talking about. What do you do to *prevent* the next medical disaster?

Here is an even more telling example: a patient goes in for a physical examination. His blood pressure is 194/94, and his physician diagnoses him with hypertension. No questions are asked about what medications the patient has been taking (decongestants for a cold, which will raise blood pressure), and he is simply put on a diuretic. Now putting a patient on a diuretic for high blood pressure is not a bad choice—in fact, it is probably the national standard. Nonetheless, when that patient comes back and his numbers are lower, we doctors feel as though we are MD's. Yep, you got it: Minor Deities. We have not done anything other than simply lower numbers. We have never asked the question, "Why is the patient hypertensive?" We have never considered other preventative solutions.

When the patient returns and the numbers are lower, if we have the time (and wouldn't that be nice in today's age of medical care!), the physician might take the time to ask the patient, "How are you feeling overall? Is everything else okay?" That's not something you really want to ask in a doctor's office because the job is to move patients through. Invariably, patients have lots of issues they would like to talk about—or better yet, be *taught* about. But if, in fact, the physician asks this gentleman about other problems, the patient might tell the physician that he noticed he is also impotent and ask if that relates at all to the high blood pressure? "Yes," responds his physician, "lots of male patients have erectile dysfunction with high blood pressure as well as diabetes. But it's no problem, though; let's give you the latest copy of Playboy wrapped up in a blue pill—V———." And the blue pill has taken off like wildfire! We still don't ask the question, "Why are patients impotent, and why do they need that blue pill?" It's just easier to write the prescription because the pill works.

So let's bring that patient back in 6 more weeks, but this time, let's do some blood work. The standard blood work on this patient shows that his blood sugar is now 134. For most physicians, that is above the 126 limit for diagnosis of diabetes, but that's okay because we have another pill called Glucophage. It is actually a very wonderful medication and used extensively for diabetics. I use it myself. Nonetheless, we now have a patient who came in for a physical examination, and he is leaving with three different medications. Yet we still have never asked the proper questions to find the root cause of why? *Why* does he have high blood pressure? Why were pills the *first* solution? And even if the pills were truly appropriate, why were they prescribed without any lifestyle changes? Where's the symphony? (Oh, and by the way, the diuretic can cause erectile dysfunction and elevated blood sugar.) There has just got to be a better way, and there is. I'm sorry that healthcare hasn't caught up yet.

It is really important to change this paradigm of mental error in the United States. This *should* be done by practicing physicians and healthcare providers, but it can also be done by you. For the average person, the day usually goes smoothly with an occasional disaster thrown in for excitement. Most evenings or casual times are spent reviewing the highlights of the day or week. And guess what? That week has turned into a month, 6 months, and yes, even years. What changes have people made during those days that will make them "better today than yesterday"? That is the problem! We just *don't*. We get caught up in living, and living is all-consuming.

After a medical emergency, we often make those quick mental promises: "I am going to cut back on my alcohol, that's for sure. And I think I'm going to start going to the gym. I am paying that monthly fee, but I hardly ever have a moment to get there." Throw in any type of self-encouragement and promises that you want; odds are that a week later you will have forgotten the pain and agony, and you will be right back to ordering a pepperoni pizza. (Not that there is anything wrong with a pepperoni pizza once in a while!) The point is that you will most likely be right back in your lifestyle without much change until the next disaster happens. You see, the problem with this paradigm is that in the United States today, as I've already mentioned, we go from medical disaster to medical disaster. It is that space in between disasters that I work on; and hopefully, you will too. That is the space where the stress is and where the lack of sleep, smoking, excess appetite, lack of activity program, and the lack of daily commitment produce the next medical disaster. I am going to try to convince you that there is a better way, but it does require a choice for change every day. It can be as simple as an index card, but it has got to be every day. Sorry.

This is probably a good time to bring up a dose of reality. Despite our best efforts, we are all going to die. Sorry, folks. I know that nobody likes to read that or hear it or have it be enforced, but it is absolutely critical to know. It does not matter how much wrinkle cream you use or how many supplements you are pouring in. The bottom line is that we are going to die. Now here is the good news: you can choose how to die or what medical care you would like in a given situation or emergency. Everyone should complete and always carry a copy of an advance directive expressing his or her wishes. There is a sample document in the appendix of this book, and copies are also available in every hospital setting.

Every state has its own requirements and terminology for living wills and advance directives. Many states require the forms to be notarized; some like Florida require other forms too. For your benefit, I have provided a copy of the basic documents that are accepted in Florida and many other states, courtesy of Project Grace (www. projectgrace.org). In addition, Project Grace has an excellent Q&A section. In order to protect yourself and ensure your wishes will be met, you should discuss this process with a physician and your family.

Don't leave this process up to your spouse; it's too much of a burden. During a crisis, family members will always say "Do everything you can, doctor!" But the fact of the matter is that there are situations where futile care is absolutely inhumane and just plain wasteful. We spend 55 cents out of every healthcare dollar on futile care—monies spent in a situation where the patient will not be better for that care. It may, and in most cases will, prolong the agony. Death is not to be feared. Death is an exciting next trip. Try not comparing it to a Disney Cruise. Nope, Disney could not compete with this voyage. It is exciting, unknown, and guaranteed to be the ride of your life!

~~~~~~~~~

"Lies, lies, I can't believe the words you say!"
—The Knickerbockers

This is a great lyric from the '60s, but it has much more meaning today. Back in the '60s, there were still lots of lies; but if you were a politician or a physician and you told lies, you were often caught, plain and simple. Nowadays, it's not so much about trying to find the lies as it really is about trying to find the truth. From six-pack abs to penis enhancers, we are deluged with health promises. If you delve into these promises, however, they turn out to be lies, or at best half-truths. And yet, the basic truths of healthy living from yesteryear still hold firm.

~ Eat less.

~ Lose weight.

~ Exercise sanely.

~ Get eight hours of sleep.

~ Drink eight glasses of water a day.

These guidelines have not changed since the beginning of writing prescriptions, and they still hold true today. All of them will help you stay healthier. But now you have promises from your doctors, your television, and, most specifically, from pharmaceutical companies. We have many varieties of pills being advocated by doctors on T.V. in nicely starched white coats. I do not wear a white coat anymore because, if you are working, they get dirty (take that any way you want). But what if you want your cholesterol lowered, your mood raised, you need to sleep, or you need to stay awake? We've got pills for all of that. On average, a 75-year-old who would like to transition to an assisted living facility will be carrying in his or her little brown bag 13 medications with Lord knows how many interactions, side effects, and deleterious daily risks. In fact, over 105,000 people die from medication each year.

Interestingly, we also have six different products for erectile dysfunction for men. Guess what gender predominates in pharmaceutical companies? And there are no new drugs coming out for disasters such as cystic fibrosis, Alzheimer's, or a host of other orphan diseases that we just don't like to talk about. Unfortunately, healthcare is all driven by potential profits. Okay, so you get it. We are trying to find the truth amidst creative marketing and commercialism. Where the heck does the truth lie? Well, these personal aphorisms sum up my entire view of truth:

~ Daily pleasure can be encouraged and prompted by the illusions presented by marketing.

~ Absolute happiness depends upon truth.

Today, it seems as though everyone—pundits, priests, politicians, and even parents—believes that the national anthem in America is: "Everyone is entitled to their own opinion!" And, of course, they are right. Opinions are free, but you get what you pay for, which brings me to a third aphorism:

~ Everyone is entitled to their own opinion, but not their own facts (or truth).

We need to delve into the facts about everything presented to us through our literature, our media, and our friends and family. It's so much easier to believe that by spending $19.95, I am going to have ripped abs or become the lover of the millennium. It's a lot harder to say to one's self, "Yeah, probably not going to happen in my lifetime." Some things are just not factual. For instance, I will never dunk a basketball. It just won't happen. Schneider genes keep me out of the Globetrotters' training camp, but I will still go watch them play.

Part of the problem with truth in medicine is that doctors often do not know it. They are trapped by the sales information from gorgeous pharmaceutical reps. (My apologies to those reps that are male, but you are probably seen as gorgeous by our female physicians.)

For example, statins are perhaps the most widely prescribed medication in the United States today—statins are the medications that lower your "cholesterol." Interestingly, "cholesterol," the word itself, comes from "chole," meaning liver, and "sterol," a derivative of "steroid." If you take the cholesterol molecule itself and place it over a steroid molecule such as cortisone, they look almost identical. Cholesterol, by the way, is made in your liver; it's not snake venom. Is cholesterol a poison? I think not. The master planner does not have you making poisons. Cholesterol is naturally occurring and is not another name for Lee Harvey Oswald or Al Capone.

Let's get back to the drugs. There seems to be a national crusade to annihilate cholesterol with statins. Cholesterol is your source of hormones, and you can't live without it. Yup, sure sounds like something we should eradicate! Or maybe not! And what are some of the side effects of these liberally prescribed statins? Are you ever told of the loss of cognition or mental abilities that can accompany statins? The association with Alzheimer's? The association with breast cancer? The high association with muscle and joint pains that could be eliminated by simply using a supplement called CoQ10? No, I do not think you are ever told about those. By the way, do those supplements work better than niacin, which is a B vitamin, or red yeast rice? Can an appetite program and an activity program help? Yes. The point is that there is a natural way to manage cholesterol. And that is the truth!

Change is possible. Now that obvious statement carries with it a burden. I might add that change is possible but very difficult. As I've said before, it really does require baby steps. If it is a question of your personal appetite, for instance, it needs to be minimal baby step changes. Perhaps start by going from 2,000 calories a day down to 1,800. But don't think that you can survive by going from 2,000 calories a day down to 800. It is just not sustainable. But change does require a daily commitment, and Yogi was right: "If you do not make a change from your direction, you will end up where you are going." If you are sitting in my office, it's not my responsibility to tell you what to do to be healthy. It *is* my responsibility to teach you about the most up-to-date science and research that can help you make your own decisions about your health and wellness.

In order to best navigate this decision-making process, I highly recommend a wellness checkup every year, as opposed to a more traditional annual medical checkup (most of the time I don't even recommend those unless you have complaints). A wellness checkup is different. It is not going to take just fifteen to twenty minutes—it is an hour or two hours, one-on-one with a physician who cares and is willing to look at the entire physical, social, neurological, and cognitive energy aspects of your life. It utilizes very specific and sophisticated labs to determine those impending processes that are so seldom looked for. And hopefully, that physician will contract with you. That means that you both take responsibility for your healthcare. Yeah, those weren't just nice phrases; they really impose a specific challenge. You cannot expect your physician to be watching your meals or waking up in the morning to encourage you to exercise. It really has to come from your heart and be a commitment to giving yourself a gift that has been long overdue.

A thorough wellness evaluation should include measures of your neurotransmitters, which are hormone-like substances in your brain that keep you stable, sleeping, healthy, happy, not craving foods, etc. Neurotransmitters are the message senders of your mind—they can be thought of as e-mail, Twitter, and Facebook all rolled into one. They have scientific names like serotonin, GABA (gamma-amino butyric acid), dopamine, and glutamate. Don't let those big names scare you; they are simply substances that help to balance your brain as well as your body. Yes, it is all in your head! (Sorry, but I had to use that "all-in-your-head" line because of a patient of mine who had multiple sclerosis and severe fibromyalgia {pain elicited in most of the muscles of the body}. She had been seen by three physicians, and they had all confirmed that her complaints, yes, you guessed it, were "all in her head." She had a drawer full of antidepressants that she had been prescribed. None helped—not the doctors or the pills!) There will be an entire chapter on neurotransmitters later in this book. So hang on to your "itchies" to jump ahead. We will get there.

It's worth mentioning that the world of medicine is changing rapidly. Expect changes in the future that will absolutely knock your socks off. We are talking about nanotechnology—or the use of microscopic machines that can enter the bloodstream and literally perform microsurgery to unblock clots. Today you can swallow a pill, and it will photograph your entire intestines. This technology is available today and doesn't necessarily obviate the need for colonoscopy, but it sure is a nice addition and easy to swallow! Every pun intended.

Stem cells are now available and have already proven to have absolutely unlimited potential. There is research going on right now that involves injecting stem cells into the heart for the purpose of increasing cardiac muscle strength. They can also be used to create new blood vessels in the heart and to augment damaged coronary arteries. How about something as benign as injecting stem cells under the scalp for hair growth?! Yep, all being done as you read.

Regenerative medicine is a field and specialty now of its own. A segment of cells can be taken from you, sculpted, and fabricated in a laboratory, producing a brand new bladder. That is already being done for children born without a bladder. What a change in their lives! The list goes on and on. The technology today is absolutely "faster than a speeding bullet." An on-top-of-it physician could spend half of his week just keeping up with the changes in research taking place; and in 6 months, he or she would have still fallen behind. Unfortunately, with the current time constraints, existing paradigms, and insurance requirements, most doctors do not have half a week to keep up with all of these changes, let alone the time to teach their patients and advocate the patient's involvement with a full wellness program.

So is your physician important? Is your input and decision making critical? Of course, yes. But how remains the issue. This will require a "you" transition—changing from the recipient of a physician's care to the conductor of your own health and wellness symphony. This may require debating with your physician or even searching for a more compatible physician for yourself and your family, and it certainly will require your active education. Thankfully, you've already gotten started—you're reading this book after all. Let's keep learning.

CHAPTER 5

Ain't No Such Thing as a Bad Food. ...Just Too Much of It

"Make food your medicine."—Quoted by a
lot of really smart guys and gals, and I agree.

So this is where we get to the nitty gritty about an appetite
program. Notice I did not say **DIET.** The first three letters
of that word scare just about everybody off, and what you do not need
is another diet book. You also do not need a number of chapters with
how-to recipes. I'm no chef. I don't have any tarragon on my herb
shelf. My herbs are salt, pepper, mustard, and ketchup.

Instead, I am going to tell you about an appetite program that
works for me and works for most of my patients. It is simple; and most
importantly, it is completely adaptable to you. For example, if I mention scrambled eggs in the morning and you cannot stand eggs, switch
it out to some of the options you do like. How about tuna and salsa?

When I see and hear about all the diet information and pills out
there, talk about an apology that needs to be made! I would not even
know where to begin with remorse for the information that we as physicians, clinicians, health care providers, and endorsers of infomercials

have given to you all. Have you ever known of a topic where there is so much confusing and diametrically opposed information? Mea culpa, mea culpa. (Old Latin training—translation: My fault, my fault.)

There have been approximately 1.1 gazillion books written about appetite and weight loss; and holy mackerel, what a great business! Weight loss and weight gain and more weight loss and more diet books and more pieces of equipment and more health products and more diet foods and more—well, you get the picture. I mention all of this because most diet and exercise books, infomercials, gyms, ill-informed doctors and nurses, insurance companies, pharmacies, and pharmaceutical companies have given us, in the vernacular from the Bronx, a crock.

What we are looking for—you *and* me—is that truth. And the truth is that diet and exercise just does not work as a prescription. Do any of these diets work? Nope—including this one. So I am going to teach you a simple and down-to-earth approach that will work even when this book is sitting on a shelf. Now I promised I would not get too scientific, but there are some facts that you just have to know first.

The Facts

Getting to an ideal weight, plus or minus five pounds, can be done in a variety of ways. Starvation is not one of them. Most people think that going from 150 pounds to 140 is quality weight loss. Not necessarily so. From my standpoint, it needs to be *fat loss*. Is there any other kind? Yes; when you simply look at diet ads and decide that you are going to lose 20 pounds in two weeks, you are going to lose muscle and water. That has to come back, and you will gain that 20 pounds back (as fat) and then gain a little more. It is fat loss that we are looking for, and that comes down to losing somewhere between 1 and 1½ pounds per week. So if you need to lose 60 lbs., do you feel a little panicked that it may take 40 weeks or more? I'm sorry, but that's the truth. Here's a little pearl that nobody mentions in any of those weight loss advertisements: what is the biggest risk from rapid weight loss (e.g., 30 pounds in a month, 60 pounds in 3 months, etc.)? Is it constipation, fatigue, or depression? No, it's death. That's right, I said death. And we, as physicians, really don't have a clue why that happens. But the fact is it does, and it's very seldom mentioned. Let me reiterate that fat loss is the goal for the prevention of cancer, diabetes, coronary artery disease, stroke, and dementia. Those disease entities are the risk of excessive fat. Your goal for fat loss may be looking great in a Speedo or bikini, but fat loss requires a daily lifestyle change for disease prevention. Safe and sane fat loss is steady—it is not a quick process. But it is sustainable; and, if done correctly, it will result in a healthier you. If it's just a fast 30 lbs. weight loss you're looking for, we can surgically remove a leg. How can it be done steadily and sanely? I am going to give you some ideas on that.

So from now on, weight loss should be defined as fat loss. You don't want to lose muscle, and you don't want to lose a tremendous amount of water. You do want to lose fat. How are we going to accomplish that? We're going to turn your car (body), which now runs on sugar, into a car that runs on fats and proteins. But first, some more fun (and not-so-fun) facts.

If you take 100 patients and put them on any commercial weight loss program that requires eating cardboard or paper mache; and if they stick to it, 75% of them will lose weight. Well, sign me up, you might say. Not so fast, Kimosabe. Let's look at the 75 patients who lost weight three years later. After those three years have passed, how many of them have gained back the weight they lost or are heavier than they were before starting the diet? 94%! Amazing. Is that absolutely true? Unfortunately, yes.

By the way, I should mention that about 10% of the population can eat anything they want and still not gain weight. They have a number of hormone-balancing and neurotransmitter paradigms that simply work. It is important to note, however, that you can be very skinny and still be very unhealthy. That is an absolute fact. Some skinny patients can have weakened coronary artery disease.

On the other end of the spectrum, here's another not-so-fun fact: In the United States, approximately 74% of us are currently either overweight or obese.

What weight should you be? Well, there are thousands of charts for that, but I keep it fairly simple. You get 100 pounds for being 5 feet (60 inches) tall. For every inch over that, you can have between 6 and 7 pounds. So if you are 5 feet 8 inches, your ideal weight should be somewhere between 150 and 155 pounds. If you were 6 feet (72 inches) tall, to find your ideal weight, you would give yourself 100 pounds for your first 5 feet (60 inches). You would then add 6×12 (for the additional 12 inches you would be over 5 feet), or 72 pounds. That would mean that your ideal weight would be 172 pounds.

This is where most of my male patients usually start beating the floor: "Only 172 pounds, Doc?! I haven't weighed that since I was a senior in high school!" Well, I'm sorry. I do not make up the rules; I can just tell you the facts. At 10 to 15 pounds above your ideal weight, you are at higher risk for coronary artery disease and diabetes, and that is just the plain fact. It may be that you decide 172 is just not right for you at 6 feet and that you really feel better and can maintain 185 pounds without a whole lot of initial stress in your life. Fine; 185 it is. Blood pressure is okay? Blood sugar is okay? Lipid panel is okay? Fine; then, let's stay at 185. If you aren't well or you are creeping up on diabetes, 10% weight loss is all it will take to start bringing that back into normal. And 10% is not that tough to do. By the way, women get this completely. Most seem to know exactly what their ideal weight should be within 5 pounds. I do not know what it is about women; maybe it is the hormone factor or maybe they are just smart. But they can always tell me within about five pounds of where they should be and usually they are spot on.

Weight loss, by the way, means losing 3,500 calories for 1 pound. When we talk about activity and exercise in the next chapter, you will see how absurd it is to try to run that pound off. If you are under 40, lucky you. Your hormones are balanced. You can run and jump and play soccer, and you certainly will lose weight. Unfortunately, most of us over 40 do not have that advantage. I can run a marathon and not lose a pound. And that is the truth. (The average 55-year-old marathoner has a net loss of 1,600 calories per race, not 3,500—that's only ½ pound for an entire marathon!) To be fair, it is possible to lose some caloric weight through regular activity, but it would require exercise 7 days a week, 7 hours a day, at a heart rate 70% of your maximum. Talk about crazy. So what are we going to do to lose this weight? Well, I'm going to get to that, I promise; but first, I'm going to dazzle you with some more facts.

Just as for many other diseases, we do have some genetic susceptibility concerning our weight and the serious challenges it can cause. "Why did Dad get cancer and my sister diabetes, and I didn't?!" Is it genetic? The fact that we have only a 20% susceptibility for disease based on our genes, as I've mentioned, means that 80% of health issues come from environment and what we do to ourselves. We bombard ourselves with toxins every day. These are internally absorbed pollutants such as PCPs, DDT, pesticides, and nicotine. Ah, cigarette smoke; cigarette smoke is a form of stimulant that you and your body absolutely need, once addicted. I am going to show you how to change that. As for other toxins, you've got carbon monoxide, alcohol, high sugars—the list goes on and on. The point is that these are stressors, all of which enhance the internal conflict that creates inflammation within our body. Even when we are eating well, we annihilate our body with certain fats that are less than ideal (as opposed to good ones like Omega 3 fatty acids), and we are putting icing on the cake, so to speak.

Despite this, most of us survive into our seventies! When you throw in viruses, bacteria, car accidents, and just downright stupidity on our part, it is amazing any of us survive into our teens, but we do. So take heart and realize that the big picture here is to simply try to decrease as many of those toxins as possible. With a few sane changes, you will be enjoying a healthy life well into your latter years, each day finding yourself better than yesterday.

Before we talk about specifics on appetite, it is really important to understand why we have cravings. We are actually driven by our neurotransmitters and hormones to eat that which we crave. That's right; I am saying that in many, many cases, we *have* to eat what we do. I will often have a patient come in and he or she will say, "Well, I do admit that I had some chocolate cake last night." There is almost always a look of shame or amusement on his or her face. My answer is always, "Good for you. You sure needed it." And I mean that. In fact, we do need most of those things that we crave and those things that have become habit forming and even necessary to function. I am going to explain a little later why someone who has 2 or 3 cups of coffee in the morning HAS to have it—that's right, I said HAS to. Without it, without that caffeine, they would literally fall back into bed and never make it through the day.

Wellness 101

So this is the general picture of Wellness 101 for you. Notice that on the right, I have listed a number of stressors. I purposely left out your boss and your teenager who decided that a tongue piercing would look wonderful for his graduation picture; but certainly, emotional stressors are huge. The point is that many of these stressors result in an increased intake of sugar (for comfort). When sugars are absorbed into your blood stream, they will attach to protein molecules. This process has a big fancy name called glycation, but it can be pictured as forming a bowling ball with spikes. That "spiked bowling ball" then rolls down your arteries and into the little small ones in your brain and into the larger ones around your heart and everywhere else. We know that this causes an inflammatory response throughout the body.

But inflammation's not such a big deal, right? Take a couple aspirin or ibuprofen and call me in the morning—but not so fast. What does inflammation cause? Damn near everything! Oh, you mean it's more

Stress = Inflamation, which causes...

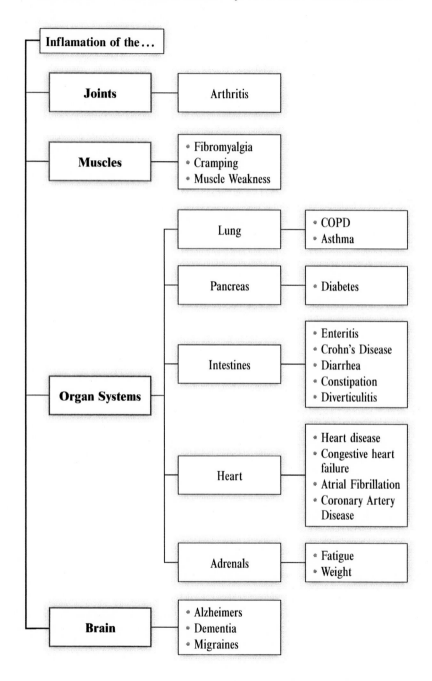

Inflamation of the...

Joints — Arthritis

Muscles —
* Fibromyalgia
* Cramping
* Muscle Weakness

Organ Systems

Lung —
* COPD
* Asthma

Pancreas —
* Diabetes

Intestines —
* Enteritis
* Crohn's Disease
* Diarrhea
* Constipation
* Diverticulitis

Heart —
* Heart disease
* Congestive heart failure
* Atrial Fibrillation
* Coronary Artery Disease

Adrenals —
* Fatigue
* Weight

Brain —
* Alzheimers
* Dementia
* Migraines

...Everything!

than just a sprained ankle? Yup. Literally, diabetes is inflammation of beta cells in the pancreas; cancer is inflammation of the nucleus of the cell; coronary artery disease is inflammation of the lining of coronary arteries; and Alzheimer's/dementia is an inflammation of glial cells in the brain that transmit impulses (or knowledge). Believe it or not, the list goes on. In fact, you want a couple more? Asthma is inflammation of the bronchial tubes in the lungs, and hypertension is inflammation causing spasm of small arteries that raise blood pressure.

Now you get the picture; but since this concept is so important, I will restate it in another way. A person is driven to eat comfort foods, usually high in sugar, when they are stressed. That sugar combines with available protein to form "spiked bowling balls," which reach every part of the body via the bloodstream. Everything they touch causes an inflammation response—the root cause for just about every disease.

The big picture here, as how stresses relate to appetite and sugar cravings, is that high levels of stress and stressors lower levels of neurotransmitters—those message senders in your brain that we've talked about. Neurotransmitters, when they're balanced, allow you to be in a Zen-like state. Getting fired seems like a relief (and opportunity) rather than a disaster. Rather than reaching for a .45 automatic, elevated neurotransmitters let you focus on the concept of "what a great opportunity this is to go back to school the way I wanted to" or "this move is going to push me into doing what I really wanted to do in life." Whatever it is that allows you to move forward and progress and be "better than yesterday" is driven by neurotransmitters in harmony.

Lower levels of neurotransmitters make us feel like poop and crave sugar. After a very stressful day, after coming home and sitting at the table and being asked if you would like a piece of cheesecake, you would reply, "No, not a piece. I'll take the entire pie!" And you probably will.

Neurotransmitters definitely control our cravings, our moods, and our ability to focus. When your level of neurotransmitters is low, then sugar, alcohol, caffeine, and resistance training (yep, something good) will raise them up. Simple sugar is a roller-coaster. A Milky Way bar will zoom your neurotransmitters to the top briefly; but those levels will be low again in about 45 minutes, leaving you with cravings for even more sugar. The more you eat because of those cravings, the more inflammation you have and the fatter you get. Lifting weights, however, will keep your neurotransmitters up for about 6 to 8 hours before they start to drift back down. Given the choice, resistance training works much better.

The truth is even doctors who know about the rollercoaster can't resist doling out the quick-fix that is sugar. Imagine a child who scraped his knee and is crying. The physician comes in and says oops, looks like we will need a tetanus shot and some (in my day) merthiolate. Oh boy, did that ever sting! So now we have a child who is in the office crying and screaming, and his neurotransmitters have dropped tremendously as his stress levels and his inflammation levels take off like an Apollo space craft. What do you think will cool his jets? Push ups? Coffee? Broccoli? Or a lollipop!? Remember, lollipops taste great. They have lots of sugar and are also rapidly absorbed. Bye bye, tears.

That was then; this is now. My wife and I adopted our daughter Ellie from China, and she goes to the pediatrician for her annual shots. After the shots, there is the usual sobbing, and guess what—she does *not* get a lollipop! It turns out that in today's modern age of technology, lollipops take too long. You do have to suck on them, and they do have to be absorbed. Is there anything faster? Yes! Pediatricians now are smart enough to have a freezer, and they keep colored sugar water in plastic tubes in that freezer. The child picks the color, and the top plastic is cut off. Then, it is just a matter of squeezing that delicious sugar water in as fast as you can. Ask my daughter. There is nothing better. Plus, I guess it is good for business on the pediatrician's behalf. Nobody likes to send a crying child out into the waiting room. Ahhh, the business of medicine.

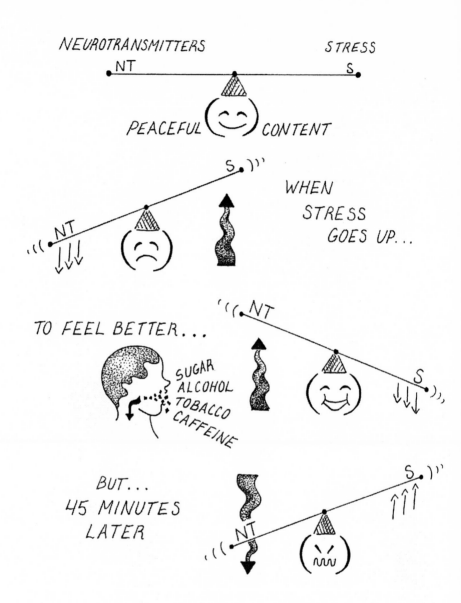

You can see how neurotransmitters play a huge role in how you feel and act, especially when it comes to an appetite or fat-loss program. It's obvious that if you want to lose weight or be on an appetite program that has a healthier bent, you've got to have your neurotransmitters stabilized. I am going to show you some easy ways to do that. Suffice it to say, for now, that increasing sugar loads ultimately decreases those neurotransmitters far more quickly than anything else.

Unfortunately, it takes a while to get out of the sugar consumption routine. The problem with the damn sugar is that it just plain tastes good. And that is a tough habit to break, but realize that having neurotransmitters elevated is what we *want* to have happen and what we *need* to have happen. When those neurotransmitters are depleted, your body says it HAS to have comfort food—potato chips, ice cream, bread, pasta.

The analogy that I often give to my patients is one of ending a triathlon. Now I like to run triathlons every so often; but truth be told, I really stink at them. I probably hold the gold medal nationally for being the worst triathlete. The typical end of a triathlon for me is finding everybody and even the finish line already gone—no exaggeration. All the other people are usually done an hour before I get there. Now to my analogy: imagine, if you will, that I am completely spent, physically and emotionally, in that parking lot. I look and see three tents still remaining. Under the first tent is my wife in a Victoria's Secret outfit. Under tent number two, the chef is barbequing grilled chicken and shrimp, and I can absolutely taste the flavors through my nostrils as they compete for the air that I am sucking in now because of my dilapidated state. And in tent number three, there is a large basin of ice-cold mountain water. What do you think I am going to crawl for? Yes, this is a MENSA test. I HAVE to have water. Sure, I may give my wife a nice wave and say thanks for the support and mumble out a request to the chef that I would love some of that "to go" in one of those Styrofoam containers, but I desperately need water—and NOW!

Well, it is no different with neurotransmitters and the needs that we have because of stressors. So if we're going through a day in which we have had high sugars, diet sodas, chips, coffees, and hosts of other inflammations, then by the time we sit down at night, our level of stress, physiologically, is extremely high. Given the choice of lasagna or chicken pieces for dinner, we are going to go for lasagna. Dessert? For me, that wouldn't be a question. I would take a double scoop of Häagen-Dazs. I love the full feeling, bloatedness, and comfort I get as a result. And where are my neurotransmitters? That's right. They are now somewhere around Pluto, but let's not relish in that for too long because they will be somewhere around Antarctica in about 45 minutes and stay there. Add bloating, belching, and heartburn to that, and I am in for a heck of a lousy night!

Here's another important fact: When you eat a candy bar, which is pure sugar, it will raise your insulin. Who cares? I do, and so should you. When my insulin goes up, and when your insulin goes up, it absolutely performs just as it was meant to and has worked for thousands of years: it makes fat. Plain and simple. That is insulin's primary purpose. It goes up in response to sugar (or carbohydrates) and does not allow the breakdown of fat (lipolysis). So every time that chocolate bar goes in, whatever else you consume, along with the chocolate bar, is going to be fat. We really want our energy to be utilized by muscle because muscle burns sugar.

Please, do not get lost here, because it does tend to get a little confusing:

Sugar in = insulin up = everything else that is consumed becomes fat.

Now that does not mean you cannot have carbohydrates, but they absolutely need to be on the low scale. To emphasize the point, here is a little quiz. I'll put you on an island with lots of water and three types of items to eat: protein, fats, and sugars. Please note, the majority of

Sugar: The Fat-maker

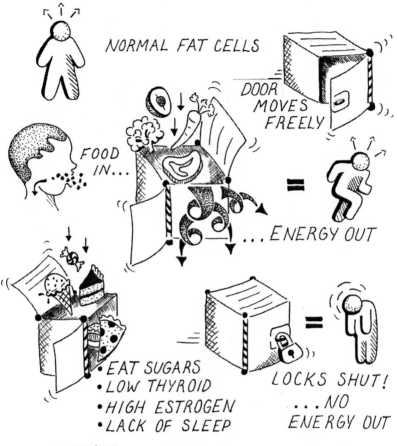

NORMAL FAT CELLS

DOOR MOVES FREELY

FOOD IN...

= ...ENERGY OUT

• EAT SUGARS
• LOW THYROID
• HIGH ESTROGEN
• LACK OF SLEEP

LOCKS SHUT! ...NO ENERGY OUT

THEREFORE... FOOD UTILIZATION IS HAMPERED

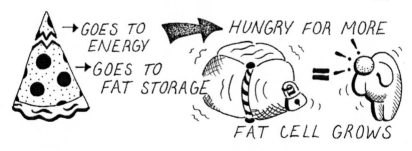

→ GOES TO ENERGY

→ GOES TO FAT STORAGE

HUNGRY FOR MORE

= FAT CELL GROWS

WHAT UNLOCKS CELL TO LOSE FAT?
• TESTOSTERONE   • EXERCISE
• THYROID   • ↓STRESS
• KETONES • PROTEINS • SLEEP

everything you eat has protein, fats, and/or sugars associated with them. So here we are on this island with those items, and I take every single bit of fat out of your diet. That includes butter, eggs, cheese, even the fat that is in meat. Let me take it out. How long will you live? About eight months! Now what if I did the same thing with proteins? What if I took all of the fish, chicken, meat, and such out of your diet—how long would you live? About ten months, and then you die. You must have fats and proteins, and you must ingest them to stay alive. Now let me ask you this important question: What if I took every single bit of sugar out of your diet? That's right, every bit of carbohydrates—I mean fruits, pies, cakes, cookies; if I took all of those sugars out of your diet, how long would you live? The answer is forever. You have no need for the consumption of sugars. Your body will make sugar and do it easily from protein. You utilize fats and their breakdown products, ketone bodies, for energy. That's pretty amazing when you think about it. Astonishing, but true.

How many grams of carbohydrates does a person need each day? In general, no more than 50–75 grams of carbohydrates total—that's net carbohydrates. To calculate net carbohydrates, look on the box and find out what the carbohydrates are. Then subtract the amount of fiber. That's the net amount of carbohydrates. *If you're an insulin diabetic or a Type I diabetic, stay at 20–40 grams per day.*

Another concept we need to address is the thin man or woman inside an obese or overweight person—or the very, very emaciated, starving person on the inside who is fat on the outside. See the diagram. Fat cells that store the energy of sugars cannot release them as energy when you need them. They remain as fat. So you eat more sugar because some of it is needed for energy. Thus, we eat more and more sugar, more and more carbohydrates, and we get fatter and fatter. Don't believe me? The big low-fat craze of the 1970s continues to this day. So we lowered the fat in any food that usually has fats, proteins, and sugars. If we lower the fats, then we must raise the sugar. It's like a water balloon; if you squeeze one part, the other part goes up. So when you squeeze down fats, up go the sugars. Hence, low-fat yogurt, low-fat ice cream, and other low-fat foods mean higher sugar. Higher sugar means increased insulin, and increased insulin means energy is not going to come out of the fat cells because the little doors are not going to open when insulin is high. It's just that simple, just that vicious, and just that cyclical.

So what can we do?

CHAPTER 6

Nutrition: The Letterman Principle

"The opposite of success isn't failure;
it's name-dropping." —Anny Mous

*D*espite what is force-fed to us in the media, there is no single pill to resolve weight gain or to cause permanent fat loss. It really does require a symphony and a defined commitment every day. Are we going to be perfect? Of course not! Chocolate chip cookies taste too darn good. But we can limit what we eat, and we can counterbalance our slips and stumbles by utilizing a symphonic approach. I love what I now call the Letterman principle. Before I went to sleep one night, I was watching *The Late Show with David Letterman* like I often do. His guests that evening were a nutritionist and a well-known physician/health advocate. The two guests proceeded to show Dave nutritious meal after nutritious meal that were displayed on a table. They had all the standards that we've come to know such as broccoli, spinach, kale, and salads galore. A couple of dishes had Brussels sprouts, and some had bok choy. Each had been cooked to perfection by master chefs and was, I'm sure, delicious. Their point to Dave was that all of us should eat accordingly. I don't disagree, but I fully agree with Dave's response. He pulled out from under the table a hot fudge sundae that was dripping with syrup. He politely wished his guests good luck, but he suggested that they couldn't win the battle because his hot fudge sundae was just—damn delicious. (And more importantly, that kind of food makes you feel good.) So can we ban the 31 flavors of Baskin-Robbins' ice cream? Can we burn down all the Krispy Kremes? Or pull Hostess cupcakes off the shelves? Or bury all of the pizza parlors? Of course not! And it's also important to know that such goodies are not evil. They are just foods with high fat, high sugar, and high salts that our bodies crave—especially under times of stress. We all have stress, and we all try to deal with it by using things like alcohol, pizza, and a host of other indulgences to fill our need. Unfortunately, these goodies also fill our love handles. Bottom line? I'm with you, Dave. Hot fudge sundaes once a week are here to stay—thank God!

Now ... HERE COME THE FACTS...

On average, the daily caloric intake for almost everyone should be between 1,000 and 1,600 calories. Normally, nobody needs to eat more than that—nobody. "But, doctor, I don't like to count calories!" I am sorry, but you must learn what 1,200 or 1,500 or 1,800 calories looks like and stick to it. "But I really don't want to do that. Isn't there something simpler?" Yes, just use a small salad plate at each one of your meals and fill it once. I don't mean you can Dagwood them (meaning stack them to the ceiling), and I definitely do not mean you should use a restaurant "feed-the-Russian-army"-style salad plate. "But there is only room for a piece of fish on a small salad plate." Well, that is your choice. Cut the fish in half and add broccoli if you like, but that is the amount of food that you should eat.

I mentioned carbohydrates as a serious intruder on our wellness, and I would like to take a moment to clarify something: carbohydrates really include just about everything other than protein (meats, fish, chicken, etc.) and fats (oils, butter, nuts). The carbohydrates that we all think about are, of course, chocolate cake, Tootsie Rolls, soda, etc. But do you think of broccoli as a sugar or carbohydrate? I smirk—it is. Now granted, it has tons of fiber, and the level of sugar in it is actually low. But it is still a carbohydrate.

In order to keep track of a food's impact, we use a scale called the glycemic index, and broccoli is fairly low on the glycemic index. This index is a measure of sugar in a food substance compared to a tablespoon of plain white sugar. So if plain white sugar is 100, broccoli might be as low as 38, but don't be fooled by that. If you eat a barrel full of broccoli, you are going to gain weight because it still has sugar—end of discussion. It's just that you can eat more broccoli than you could, for example, baked potatoes. The glycemic index of a baked potato is 81. In general, it's best to eat foods with an index under 60. By the way, the glycemic index can be downloaded on the web at www.glycemicindex.com.

It doesn't take long to go online to research the number of grams of carbohydrates an item contains. You can also look on the nutritional label in one of numerous pamphlets readily available in most food stores. Just remember to subtract the grams of fiber. An apple, for example, has roughly 22 grams of carbohydrates and 5 grams of fiber, so it has about 17 net carbohydrates. The amount of sugar, including that from carbohydrates (e.g. broccoli, fruits, and sweets), that you eat each day should never exceed 100 grams. It's best for diabetics to be at 50 grams or fewer.

The next step is to understand where you are metabolically right now. That requires a number of blood tests that need to be evaluated. They are:

~ blood count	~ hs-CRP
~ urinalysis	~ NMR (lipid panel)
~ thyroid function test	~ fasting blood sugar
~ free T-3 (thyroid)	~ hemoglobin A1c

~ estradiol level   ~ estrogen

~ free testosterone

For the absolute best evaluation, if you can afford it (though how much is your health worth to you?), I would also have saliva tests and urine tests done for serotonin, gamma, dopamine, norepinephrine, and cortisol. These are the neurotransmitters that I was speaking about earlier, and they can easily be balanced.

"Great, Doc! So all I need is a physical examination and some basic labs to get started!" Unfortunately, no. It actually starts with that commitment to change that we spoke about. The mind is probably the biggest weight loss driver that we have. When we overeat—and particularly overeat carbohydrates like cheesecake and my favorite, Häagen-Dazs ice cream—it is usually to satisfy a craving. It could be an emotional craving, or it could be a neurotransmitter craving. It might just be an energy craving. Nonetheless, handling the cravings is truly important. If your life is in chaos with your partner, your work, or your understanding of your needs, weight loss is going to be downright difficult. (Not impossible, mind you, but difficult.)

The principles of weight loss for me have to do with simplicity; so after committing to change, you should record your current weight and waist size if you haven't already.

The next step is to decide what you want. By that, I mean you need to determine what a safe goal is for you—something not too low and not too high. We have already provided the guidelines for a goal weight. To recap, you get 100 pounds at 5 feet tall and an additional 6 pounds for every inch over 5 feet. For example, if you are 6 feet tall, you get 172 pounds as a sane weight, plus or minus 5 pounds.

"But, Doc ..." No, I get it. At 6 feet, 200 pounds *may* be okay for you. The number above is just a safe guideline to keep you in a non-disease-prone weight range.

Now having determined your goal weight, multiply your goal weight by 10. That is the easiest way to determine the number of calories you can have in order to maintain a healthy weight. It sounds pretty simple on paper, but it is difficult for many people because it means counting calories. Frankly, I just cannot do that. So to make it easier, I have given you examples of what meals for a daily intake of 1,200, 1,500, and 1,800 calories looks like in the reference section of this book.

Still don't want to count calories? Looking for another way? Then, try the 60 gram, 80 gram, or 90 gram carbohydrate plan. For most men, staying under 100 carbs per day will allow them to maintain or lose weight. For women, 80 grams would be the number to try to stay below. For diabetics, try to stay under 60 grams. In the back of the book, you will also find examples of what 60, 80, and 90 gram carbohydrate appetite programs look like. The 90 gram weight loss program will help you lose weight like the others, but it's a little easier to initiate. These pathways simplify your program since instead of counting calories, you are counting the carbohydrates in the products that you are eating. Remember, items like meats, fowl, fish, and fats really have minimal carbohydrates. Since you can subtract the amount of fiber in an item as well, a piece of toast may only *count* as thirteen grams of carbohydrates even if it technically has fifteen grams, provided there are 2 grams of fiber per slice—pretty simple. It's very easy during the day to simply count the number of carbohydrates you are consuming. If the 90 gram program isn't bold enough for you, you can try the 80 or 60 gram programs for a little more rapid weight loss.

> [**Note for diabetics:** Diabetes is a toughie. Patients with diabetes have a craving for carbohydrates because although they are taking them in, the carbohydrates are stored in fat and are unable to be released for energy so they feel the craving to consume more and more. It's the same ol' starving person trapped inside the facade of an over-fed body—the starving person simply cannot get the energy that is being stored in the fat cells.

Dr. Joseph Bernstein's program is great for diabetics. Dr. Bernstein, who is, in my opinion, the diabetic practical physician extraordinaire, has a 6–12–12 program. In this program, he simply asks his patients to use 6 grams of carbohydrates for a breakfast meal, 12 for lunch, and 12 for dinner. Notice that this is *just* carbohydrates. In general, there is no restriction on the amount of protein that you can eat. If this sounds a tad like the Adkins diet, it is similar, but it allows carbohydrates. Hydrating is the only other requirement, and I suggest taking a multivitamin as well. By the way, this method is safe and absolutely works whether you're diabetic or not.]

Here is the real deal: going on a low-carbohydrate appetite program will definitely cause you to lose weight. My suggestion, though, would be that you not set a goal of 20 pound weight loss. Your goal really needs to be a commitment to a lifestyle change, not just to chucking off as much weight as possible. So what I am suggesting is that for 6 days a week, you live an appetite program using about 60 grams of carbohydrates a day. "Oops, I went to 80 or 100 today!" No big deal. The point is that this is a process—one with ups and downs. Overall, you want to maintain approximately 60 to 80 grams of carbohydrates per day, 6 days a week. "Hey, wait a minute, Doc; there are 7 days in a week." Oh, that's right. Okay, so what about Saturday? Saturday is a freebie. Have that pizza that you have been looking forward to, or have that scoop of ice cream. Why? Because they taste good! They follow the Letterman principle. And you can always have that craving during the week and put it off by saying, "You know what? I am going to have that pasta supreme pizza on Saturday." But what if that craving just gets to be too much? You know the night—that Wednesday night as the television ads show a sub sandwich after pizza after toasted roll. There is a point when I just want to cave in. I have a craving, and I need to satiate it—now!

Well, here are some of my thoughts. My first rule is this: Go ahead and cave in—just don't crash in. If you are hungry for something that is sweet, take a piece of dark chocolate and enjoy every morsel. No, I do not mean gobble it up. I mean really savor small pieces and let it melt in your mouth. You will be amazed how satisfying it is. Also, if you are feeling hungry, it usually means that you are also dehydrated. A cup of broth will work wonders, so go ahead and throw some croutons in as well. The whole point of all of this is to make your program relatively enjoyable because *it is a lifestyle change, not a diet.* It's something that you have to be able to live with.

So how hard is this? I mean, seriously! You are going to be eating somewhere between 1,200 and 1,600 calories a day, and the amount of carbohydrates that you are going to be consuming will be around 60 or 80 grams per day. Using the glycemic index (www.glycemicindex.com), you can find those carbohydrates that are lower on the index than others, and you get to have your treats as well. They are part of life, so enjoy them.

"Hey, Doc, I had a little trouble with high school algebra, and these numbers are driving me crazy. What's something I can live with if I'm out camping or in a restaurant?" Here's an easy technique for everyone, regardless of your size.

Take a look at your hand and map out your palm. Now the palm can include the thumb but not the other four fingers. That size and that thickness represents an excellent average amount of protein per meal. So if you're having scrambled eggs, have the amount that is the size and thickness of your palm. How about fish? Steak? Chicken? Same thing—enjoy the size of your palm. Now take your palm and your fingers and form a cup—just one hand now. Fill that cup with vegetables. That's the amount you can have. Make them dark green vegetables such as broccoli or asparagus and you get extra points in the nutrition derby. Now take that hand as a cup and fill it with salad. There you go—a nice, simple meal. Look at your thumb. Pretend it's hollow and fill it with salad dressing. Do you like butter? Fill your pinky with butter. Add a glass of iced lemon water and bon appetite! Notice there were no fingers to fill with french fries or mashed potatoes with gravy. That's okay; remember you still have Saturday. Feel free to enjoy the "Letterman goodies"—including ice cream. Want to keep it safe? Then whatever goodie you're adding—a donut or ice cream or cake—make it the size that will fit into the cup of your hand. It's a simpler plan than one that might require a prerequisite course of Hooked on Phonics.

Let me make a few other points that I think are critical for weight loss. There are some patients who have severe sleep apnea or a simple sleep disorder. That really has to be corrected for adequate weight loss. As I've already mentioned, if you are not getting enough sleep, you won't lose weight. If you are not sleeping well, you are in a state of sleep deprivation, resulting in high insulin levels. High insulin levels will lower your neurotransmitters, and you will absolutely feel the need to take in carbohydrates the next day. And when insulin levels are high, everything you eat actually goes to fat instead of going to energy.

"Hey Doc, what about all the exercise? And what happens when I reach my goal weight?" I'm glad you asked. First, you don't need more than 15 minutes of fun exercise a day. We'll cover activity programs in the next chapter, and I'll show you that the exercise is for hormone balancing NOT burning calories! And yup, walking or gardening counts.

Once you hit your goal weight, using low-carbohydrate protein shakes for a breakfast meal replacement works wonders for maintenance. I use them 2 or 3 times a week to maintain. Other proteins for breakfast will work as well such as turkey and cheese or chicken and salsa.

So what's the best diet? The first point is that no one diet works for everyone. The American Board of Obesity Medicine and the American Society of Bariatric Physicians currently recommend a low-carbohydrate (less than 60 grams of carbohydrates a day) appetite program. I've included an example of a meal with 60 grams of carbohydrates in the appendix. Books that describe in detail how you can eat a low-carb diet are *The All-New Atkins Advantage* and *Atkins Diabetes Revolution.* Variations on these types of programs include *The Paleo Solution,* espoused by Robb Wolf, or *The Paleo Diet* by Loren Cordain.

Regardless of the approach you choose out of the programs I've covered, there are some essential guidelines to follow to be successful with any of them. I call them the 7 S's:

~ The first S is to have a protein shake for breakfast. Find options with less than 10 grams of carbs. Matrix by Syntrax (www. syntrax.com) and shakes from Leaner Living (www.leanerliv ing.com) are delicious. Add sugar-free flavoring from www. davincigourmet.com.

~ The second S is snack. Have one mid-morning and one mid-afternoon snack. These can include chunky peanut butter, celery, cheese, tuna, chicken, or nuts (just a handful). No fruit and no breads—"If it's white, don't bite."

~ The next S is salad. A salad for lunch and dinner is fine, but watch the carbs in the salad dressing. All I need you to do is eat it on a small salad plate. That's it.

~ The next S is sports. We'll cover activity programs in the next chapter, but here's the shorthand: It might be walking, or it might be a full session at the gym. I don't care, and neither does your body. Just move your muscles to soak in damaging processed sugars.

~ The next S is supplements. There are supplements that actually help to increase your metabolism. We will discuss those later. But if you like green tea, drink it liberally throughout the day to increase your metabolism.

~ The next S is fiber. Yeah, I know—it doesn't begin with S, but I just couldn't put down "slush." We'll discuss more on fiber in just a second.

~ The last S is Saturday. Saturday is the day you can enjoy because you were doing so well on Wednesday with your 1,500 calories of high-protein diet, but now you're just dying for a slice of pizza. Go ahead; it's Saturday. You want that scoop of Hagen Daas ice cream? Go ahead—have a scoop of ice cream. You'd like a brownie? Go ahead and have a brownie. Now please understand that I'm not recommending that you have a slice of pizza with a brownie and Häagen-Dazs on top. Sound nauseating? Good—it should! But there will be cravings and foods you absolutely have to have. My dictum is to go ahead. Life is to be lived; and again, there is no such thing as a bad food—just way too much of it. As a diabetic, do I ever have my ice cream? You already know the answer. Absolutely, but never more than a scoop every week.

Now back to that fiber thing. One of the most important components of a weight loss program that is truly effective is increasing fiber. Fiber is one of the least-mentioned and certainly the most underrated of ingestions that we can consume. It is not only beneficial to your colon and small intestine, but it is very effective for weight loss as well. A daily requirement for fiber in a weight loss program is 50 grams per day total. Many of the foods that you are ingesting with fiber such as broccoli, peanut butter, and nuts are fantastic adjuncts to one's appetite program. Fiber is listed as one of the nutritional components on the packaging of just about all of the products you buy. The problem is that nobody eats two quarts of broccoli and one quart of kale per day to obtain their 50 grams of fiber. Most of us require fiber supplementation. There are numerous commercial products (Metamucil, Fiber One, etc.) that can be taken in a protein shake or by themselves throughout the day. The benefits from increasing one's fiber include weight loss, insulin control, lipid stabilization, and decreased bowel transit time (a great thing unless you are on the New Jersey Turnpike and 30 miles from the next rest stop).

And what if you want to get your children healthy too? Do not get me started on children because 35% are already overweight or obese, and the numbers are climbing faster than in the adult population. Five-year-olds are now getting diagnosed with type-2 diabetes (which is characteristically caused by being overweight/obese, meaning you aren't born with this one). This is a serious negative indicator of their future health. This is a national, cultural, social, and ethical disaster. As far as the children are concerned, unless we as adults take an active role and give our time to teaching, it will be nothing but catastrophic. That means sitting down at night and explaining the value of celery and tomatoes and chicken and fish to our children. It means growing a garden. No room? Use pots or window boxes! Also explain to your children about how a popsicle can be fun and enjoyable as a special treat once a week, but then it will absolutely beat up and punch the insides of us if we have one on a nightly basis.

When I showed 7-year-olds a baked potato, they had no idea what it was. When I showed them a squashed McDonald's French fries box, they all shouted, "French fries!" "No, it's just a box," I replied. Whether the box was full or empty, they were already trained. They all knew what French fries looked like. This insanity has got to stop, but it is going to take time and commitment on all of our parts. I know the multiplication tables are important, but for goodness' sake, health takes precedence over everything.

So what is the answer? Choose to live; be in charge! It really comes down to not letting the world take over our lives and minds (and those of our children). We are better than that. We have to be in control. A portion of the day has to be set aside to define what our meals will be. No, it will not be a drive-thru of fast foods. The kids are going to help with putting out the pickles and tomatoes and lettuce. Someone is going to be assigned to get the water with lemon as a drink. The meal will be chosen by Mom or Dad, and that will be it. "But I don't like this fish. Can I have something else?" The answer at some point, Moms and Dads, has to be, "No—broiled, baked, breaded—your choice, but fish it is!" Sound hardcore? Not really when you stop to think about it. Isn't that our primary role as parents—to teach? And what better thing to teach our children than about their health? Our children need to learn that healthy eating is not just about *what* we eat, but it's also about *how much* we eat.

I distinctly remember the only teaching I got when I was a young lad: "Eat it! There are children starving in China, and I want to see a clean plate!" I always wanted to send my lima beans off to China, but the fact is that cleaning your plate is not a reputable goal. Perhaps choosing a smaller amount to put on the plate would be a better choice. Cleaning the plate, regardless of how full we are, teaches us that being stuffed is the goal.

By the way, I now have one of those children from China—my daughter—and *she* reminds me to eat my lima beans! I guess what goes around does come around.

The Idiot's Guide to Weight Loss

Somehow I think there's someone reading this and saying, "Just shoot me. I can't take any more of this diet stuff and counting this and calculating that. Isn't there just a simple paradigm that I can use for weight loss or avoiding weight gain?" Okay, here goes. Just try drinking 16 ounces of ice water before each meal—that's breakfast, lunch, and dinner. You've got to drink it all down before you touch a morsel. Next, as I mentioned before, eat all of your meals off a small salad plate. Again, I'm not talking about the super-salad trough that you get at most restaurants; just use a plate that's about 6 inches in diameter. Half of the plate can be filled with vegetables, mostly green. The other half can be absolutely any protein that you like. Feel like a cheeseburger with extra cheese and bacon? Go for it—just don't eat any bread. Feeling healthy tonight? How about filling that half plate with salmon and olive oil? Only two things on the plate can be white: cauliflower and the plate itself. Otherwise, if it's white, don't bite. Breakfast? Fill the plate with a vegetable omelet, and yes, keep the yoke—that's no joke. The yellow is filled with heart-healthy lipids. And what about snacks? Have 2 a day that fill your cupped hand. Examples are celery, cheese, nuts, or blueberries. Craving chocolate? Go ahead and have a square of dark chocolate—and that's it. Notice there's no mention of exercising. Remember, it's great for lowering insulin and balancing hormones, but it's not very efficient at burning calories. You didn't see a lot of fruit recommended above either. Remember that fruit is sugar and should be eaten in moderation, particularly if you're diabetic. Also, always give yourself a one-meal-a-week vacation.

continued

Yep, maybe Saturday night is pizza night. Go ahead and enjoy. However, don't forget the 16 ounces of water first.

Too many numbers? Too much hassle? Too regimented? Why not try the latest researched appetite program? It's pretty simple. Pick 8 hours of your waking day (10 am to 6 pm for example) and eat approximately 1500 calories of whatever you like. The following 16 hours you'll spend sleeping, exercising, or drinking clear liquids—like coffee, water, and tea—to your heart's content. Participants of studies following this type of diet had the greatest percentage of fat loss versus other diet programs. No bologna! This simplified method has science behind it. Interested? Read *The Eight-Hour Diet* by David Zinczenko and Peter Moore. Try the *Paleo Diet* as a great lifestyle appetite program.

CHAPTER 7

Activities:
Let's Get Started

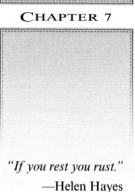

"If you rest you rust."

—Helen Hayes

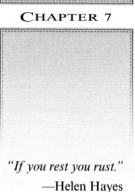otice that the topic here is not exercise; it is activity. Activities can include gardening, yoga, and even badminton. Does it also include resistance training, weights, and jogging? Of course; but what we are really going to talk about is *moving*. It doesn't have to be prescribed, and it doesn't have to be in a gym. But here is the rule: if you rest, you rust. And it does not matter how disabled you are. If you have a finger that moves, move it. So no, activity does not include meditation, even though I love meditation.

Remember that the activity is not about losing weight; it's for balancing neurotransmitters. As we've discussed, if you want to lose 1 pound, you would have to burn 3,500 calories. Now, just for grins, if you want to run that 1 pound off on a treadmill, plan on running at a level of 6.5 mph. If you have not done that recently, I can tell you that as someone who exercises every day, I could not do it for more than 3 minutes. It is really screaming; but let's just say that you and I did decide to go for it at 6.5 mph on the treadmill. How long would it take us to lose that 1 pound at that rate? 8.7 hours!! That is not a lie. Do the math for yourself. In case you want to really give yourself a thrill, try it. Let me know how that works for ya. Yeah! What are most treadmills at our houses doing right now? Holding up dresses and slacks!

So what should you do? Let's not overcomplicate things here—aerobic schmarobic. The principles for activity are fairly simple. Activity is anything that gets air moving in and out of your lungs faster. Competent exercise physiologists recommend activity that puts your heart rate in the range of 60% to 80% of your maximum heart rate. Now what is that maximum heart rate? Stay with me; I am going to have to throw in a little math here. Take 220 minus your age and then multiply that by 0.6 or 0.8. So if you are 50 years old, then the math is simply 220 minus 50, which equals 170. Multiply 170 by .6, and you get 102. (To make this easier, you can take a look at the chart on the facing page.) If you are 50 years old, 102 is the max heart rate for you to be working for during exercise. 102? Yeah, that may not seem like a heck of a lot of output for a real health benefit. But it is safe, and it will keep your heart happy with you. Heck, I can get to 102 just by walking uphill with a dog. Feeling a little more macho than that? How about 80% of your maximum heart rate? For a 50 year old, that would be 136 ($170 \times 0.8 = 136$). That's really flying. Now, my recommendation when pushing to that level is to use what are called intervals. An example would be 1 minute at 80% of your maximum heart rate and 2 minutes (or longer) at 60%. Increased heart rate/decreased heart rate is an interval pattern for a workout. And how long do you do that for? Twenty minutes. That's it—20 minutes, 6 to 7 days a week. Think you can go 30 minutes? Go for it. More than 30? I'd like to tell you to get a life; but if that's what floats your boat, give it a whirl. Whatever you do, it's important to do the interval technique since it's the safest technique for your heart.

Heart Rate Chart

Age	Low Heart Rate	High Heart Rate	Age	Low Heart Rate	High Heart Rate
30	114	152	56	98.4	131.2
31	113.4	151.2	57	97.8	130.4
32	112.8	150.4	58	97.2	129.6
33	112.2	149.6	59	96.6	128.8
34	111.6	148.8	60	96	128
35	111	148	61	95.4	127.2
36	110.4	147.2	62	94.8	126.4
37	109.8	146.4	63	94.2	125.6
38	109.2	145.6	64	93.6	124.8
39	108.6	144.8	65	93	124
40	108	144	66	92.4	123.2
41	107.4	143.2	67	91.8	122.4
42	106.8	142.4	68	91.2	121.6
43	106.2	141.6	69	90.6	120.8
44	105.6	140.8	70	90	120
45	105	140	71	89.4	119.2
46	104.4	139.2	72	88.8	118.4
47	103.8	138.4	73	88.2	117.6
48	103.2	137.6	74	87.6	116.8
49	102.6	136.8	75	87	116
50	102	136	76	86.4	115.2
51	101.4	135.2	77	85.8	114.4
52	100.8	134.4	78	85.2	113.6
53	100.2	133.6	79	84.6	112.8
54	99.6	132.8	80	84	112
55	99	132			

Now what about resistance training? Resistance training refers to lifting weights, using resistance bands, or using your body as a weight. If done properly, these techniques work not only your core muscles but your peripherals as well such as the biceps or triceps in your arms or the hamstrings or quads in your legs.

Moving quickly from one resistance activity to another means that these routines are now also aerobic activities. Resistance training is actually very, very safe when done properly. Here are a few basic safety principles that you can't go wrong with:

~ Never perform a resistance activity using a weight that you can't lift safely at least 15 times. "But, Doc, I want to look like Ahhnold." Ok, you want to lift more weight than that? Get friends to assist you.

~ Never do a full range of motion. For example, during a bench press, never bring the barbell past 12 inches above your chest. Closer than that could cost you a rotator cuff surgery.

~ During a workout session, do about 12 different *sets* of exercises—each with 15 repetitions. A repetition is a specific exercise movement, such as one squat. It is repeated a certain number of times to create a set. So 15 squats in a row is 15 repetitions in one set. Three sets of 15 squats would be a total of 45 repetitions. Wait at least 1 minute between sets. Here is an example of a workout:

> 3 sets – squats
> 2 sets – bicep curls
> 2 sets – triceps
> 3 sets – bench press
> 2 sets – pushups
> _____
> 12 total sets

~ Proper form is important, and there are a number of fantastic sources regarding the proper form for resistance training A few great places to start are www.menshealth.com and www. womenshealthmag.com. Not web savvy? Trainers are around at any local gym or YMCA, and they'll be delighted to work with you. Just remember the points above.

I recommend doing resistance training every day or nearly every day. I know what you have heard and what you're trying to say: "Don't I need to give my muscles a chance to rest?" Well, if you are going for the Mr. Universe contest, then absolutely. But if you are like me, at 67, I just want to stay toned and keep my strength up. Twelve sets of varying exercises along with 20 minutes of aerobics are all it takes. Now, if you prefer, do 12 sets one day and 20 minutes of aerobics the next. I also work some kind of stretching such as yoga into my week because I think it is not only great for the muscles that have been utilized but also for the mind. You may want to do the same.

Along with yoga, Pilates is also wonderful. We don't know why it works so well, but it sure as the dickens does. It seems to involve neurotransmitters (increasing serotonin with release of endorphins). It has a phenomenal effect on post-cardiac patients and is a mandatory part of Dr. Dean Ornish's cardiac wellness program.

As a common sense point, let me mention that it is not unusual to hear about a patient falling over from a heart attack at his desk or while jogging. But how often do you hear of someone having a heart attack while lifting weights? I never have.

Now let's put this all together in a package. Since exercise isn't gangbusters for burning calories, what really is the purpose? Well, here is what we do know about exercise:

Exercise . . .

    . . . uses some of the sugar in our bodies before it bonds with proteins. (Remember those balls with spikes we are trying to avoid?)

... lowers insulin. (Insulin helps sugar turn into fat—goodbye, love handles.)

... lowers estrogen. (Estrogen actually creates fat.)

... increases testosterone. (Testosterone decreases body fat.)

... increases thyroid hormone. (Thyroid hormone increases your metabolism and decreases stores of body fat.)

Resistance training and aerobics will absolutely balance hormones. It will, as I mentioned, lower insulin as well. One more important point about insulin: it can be very inflammatory. As insulin increases due to eating sugar or carbohydrates, it becomes less effective in putting sugar into the muscles as needed, allowing more sugar to go into our fat cells. Hello again, love handles. It's kind of like creating one beautiful painting in a day. The colors are perfect. The composition is great. If I asked you to create a thousand paintings in a day, the artwork would get sloppy, painful to look at, and none would be the kind of work you'd want to hang on your wall. Well, the same is true with insulin. The more you input sugar, the higher your insulin will go. The more insulin you have, the less effective it is. That ineffective insulin, though, does a wonderful job at inflaming everything, including coronary arteries.

Insulin also does a great job of taking whatever you eat and shoving it into your fat cells. So the whole secret there is to lower your insulin levels. Now you get it! So exercising 30 minutes a day lowers insulin levels and balances hormones (our neurotransmitters), and therein lies the beauty of exercise. Incidentally, it is the hormonal balancing that will eradicate that stubborn layer of apron fat under the tummy—also known as the omentum.

Here's another point: When I exercise, insulin goes down and sugar goes down; and to my benefit, the other hormones and neurotransmitters go up. Then why am I limited to just doing 30 minutes of exercise at one time? Why not do 10 or 15 minutes 3 times a day? To me, increasing the number of times you exercise and decreasing the amount of time at once makes complete sense, although we have no scientific data to support it. It would mean 15 minutes in the morning of jumping rope or doing stretching and yoga, 15 minutes before lunch of doing squats and push-ups against the wall at work, and then in the evening before dinner, doing some free weights, resistance training, and/or aerobics. There you have it; you have spread it out throughout the day at the points in the day when our insulin will naturally skyrocket from those wonderful things we call meals. Just seems to me to make a whole lot of sense that way; but as I told you, it is just my opinion.

Thirty minutes a day of resistance training is recommended, but I'm sure some of you are saying, "I'm too busy, Doc." Okay, do 20 minutes. "Doctor, I cannot even give you 10 minutes; I am so busy." Okay, well, here is the truth, my friend. If you haven't got 10 minutes, then get a new life! You really do have to put *you* as a priority. I'm sorry.

Want a good strategy to help make yourself exercise? It's great to have an exercise partner. Involve your partner, your friend, or a family member and do it together. People who work out together exercise more often and more consistently. If you have a child, get your child involved. My daughter Ellie works out with me at least four nights a week, and she loves it. The unfortunate part is that she wipes me out in every aspect of the exercise program we are doing each night. That is kind of intimidating because she is only eight! But that's okay; she'll be my age one day. What goes around comes around.

In the end, what is it all about? It's about TRUTH. And the TRUTH is whether we are doing 6 days a week of resistance training, 4 days a week of yoga, or 30 minutes a day of moving that one working finger, activity and movement are key instruments in the symphony of a healthy life. If you rest, you rust.

Do you want to increase your physical activity without increasing your time at the gym? Try these simple tips:

~ Park further away from your destination.

~ Take the stairs.

~ Fidget more.

~ Walk while talking on the phone.

~ Meet friends for a walk instead of a frappuccino.

~ Try out frisbee golf at your local park.

CHAPTER 8

Happiness: The Secret Lies Within, Grasshopper

"I went to a happiness conference; researchers looked very sad."

*N*ow that we've covered nutrition and activity plans, let's talk about something even more important to your well-being. It's one of the biggest problems that I see in my office. Patients come see me because of fatigue or lack of libido or weight problems. It really doesn't matter what the dilemma is. If I could cut away all of the chaff in order to get to the heart and core of my patients, I would ask one question: "What do you want most out of life?" Almost invariably the answer would be happiness. Isn't that what all of us want, to some extent, every day? And in today's society, I think all of us have learned that it does not come wrapped up in a Lexus or the newest and lightest computer. It doesn't even come in the best-looking suit or those incredibly sexy dark glasses.

Most of all, please know that happiness can only come from within ourselves. I'm sorry if that sounds like a line from David

Carradine in the old *Kung Fu* TV series, but it's true. You can't get happiness from your child's success. If you do, you are sliding down a slippery slope. When little Johnny wins first place in the freestyle swim meet, you're elated and jumping, saying, "That's my boy!" You're so excited and thrilled for him. Now, don't get me wrong. The excitement is natural, and it's great. However, is it possible to focus on explaining to Johnny how proud you are for how well he accomplished his goal, whether he took second or third or last? My point is that whether they are getting straight A's in school or straight D's with that occasional C, do we focus on the C? Are we looking for success elsewhere? Are we looking for happiness in the Lexus? The happiness we have *has* to come from within. Now, I can say that and sound like Carradine all day long, and most of my patients will dutifully nod and say, "Yes, I understand." But no, they don't; and it's a very difficult process to understand. I explain to all my patients that I don't have the master key to happiness, but that I *have* found a method that I use *every day*, and it seems to help.

I have to give a little preface so you realize that at one point in my life, I was lying horizontally on a table and looking about the color of white crystal sand. I had just come out of bypass surgery with tubes sticking out everywhere. There was a giant tube in my mouth, and I watched the bellows of the oxygenator move up and down in sync with my lungs. I had control over nothing, but I cherished the air each time the machine would pump. I've never forgotten that day, and I hope that you never have to experience it. But if you do, one of two things will happen. You'll either forget about it, or you'll never forget.

What does that have to do with happiness, you smirk? Everything. I have a mnemonic for enjoyment and happiness, and I'm happy to give it to you. You can come up with your own, or you're welcome to use mine. The mnemonic is GAGE. I use this mnemonic every single morning. Somewhere around 6:30 a.m., I roll out of bed, and I walk from my bedroom in boxer shorts. I head to my daughter's room to give her a gentle kiss for a wakeup, and I stop midway. As I look out into the backyard, I take a deep breath, and I say GAGE. Then I remember every one of those letters. It only takes about 30 seconds, but it sets my tone for the day. Every day that I forget to do it, the day turns out to be somewhat of a disaster.

(G) **The first G is give.** This G reminds me that I am to give every day in some way. I don't mean to the Red Cross or to a meaningful charity. Sure, you can do that as well, but the best way to do this step is to give to people. Which ones? The spectrum is enormous. It can start with my wife when I give her a compliment for the day. Sometimes it's hard; sometimes she wakes up and looks like the dragon lady. Nonetheless, I lie and roll over and say, "You knock my socks off, girl." My act of giving can be to the waitress who is serving me for lunch. It is so easy for me to say at the end of the meal as I hand her my payment for the check, "By the way, I've got to tell you: you did an amazingly good job, and I thank you so much." What do I get for that? A big smile. Who wins? Me. I'll bet it makes her day as well. It doesn't matter where or what you do; the opportunities are everywhere. You either connect eye-to-eye or heart-to-heart with people you meet or you don't. You're either a tourist on this planet with other people or you create an international home where everyone you meet is an opportunity to give. Now don't get me wrong. Some days I bite the side of my tongue when I meet an obnoxious character. And I'd be lying if I told you that what I do is give in those situations. I don't. I just interact. I don't need a negative anchor anywhere in my life. So I move on to my next victim to give to.

(A) **The A is for acceptance.** Acceptance is one that I learned while I was lying horizontally on that table. My son came into the Intensive Care Unit and tweaked my big toe. He came up to the side of my bed, rubbed my forehead, and gently whispered, "It's okay, Dad. This is gonna all pass." I have never forgotten those words, and they were never said more meaningfully. Indeed, the pain and the machines left, but the memory never did. Accepting whatever the disaster is today is the hardest thing that I still work on. It's very hard to try to live in the present and remember that everything will pass, but I do think it's the key to life. As a way to remember this, each day when I awaken, I lie for a moment in my bed, and I remember the feeling of my back on the mattress, my heels on the mattress, my head on the mattress, and my hands to the side. I remind myself that I will be in this pose one day for eternity. We all will die, and today may be my last day on the face of this earth. Maybe I'll be lucky and get tomorrow, but today is all I know I will have.

(G) **The second G is gratitude—gratitude for every single breath.** No, I don't remember every single breath I take, but I do recall, at least at mealtimes, a deep satiating breath to remind myself that this amazing breath is a gift to me. I remember that there was a time when the only breath I had came from a machine. So, I have gratitude for everything—gratitude for the hard times, gratitude to be out of a rice paddy in Vietnam, and gratitude for the good times like seeing all of my children and seeing my wife smile. They all have made me what I am today. I can't say enough about gratitude because I think it is the core essence for happiness. My wife and I tell each other three "thankfuls" of the day before falling asleep. Now someone reading this might say, "Yeah, but I thought this was all about my happiness, Doc," and it is. That's where the E comes in.

(E) **The E is for enjoyment.** "Yeah, that's what I'm talking about, Doc. How do I get to enjoy?" Well, it's kind of like a math formula. Do the giving, do the accepting, and do the gratitude. They add up to daily happiness. That is an absolute 100% money-back guarantee, but I'd be lying if I said it didn't take work—work in the form of realizing GAGE every single day.

Male Hormones

"It ain't that hard."

You might notice that I've put the male hormone chapter first before the female's. The reason for that is simply that guys just don't get it. I'm not sure why women do. It's probably related to menses, hormones, and the fact that they deal with it all their lives. Guys, it's going to take a while, but it's not as hard as golf, if that's your thing.

So how does it all begin for men? Well, gentlemen, until the age of about 35, your primary hormone deals with testosterone. Testosterone is a ubiquitous hormone that affects every part of your body. Now please listen to this because it's more important than who's going to win the big game. Testosterone is a hormone that primarily has receptors in the heart. Yep, I know, that was disappointing. You were thinking groin, groin, groin, weren't you? Well, the fact of the matter is the heart is maximally protected by the hormone testosterone.

In 1994, I had a heart attack and subsequently had cardiac bypass (particularly delightful). Following that trauma, I required five coronary stents (another joy!). It's 2013, and I do 15 pull-ups, 100 push-ups, and a slew of other exercising, including yoga and sculling. Cognitively, everything still seems to be working, although my wife would probably argue against that point. The fact is that 60% of testosterone receptors involve the heart. Now here comes the one you guys were waiting for—what about 35% of the receptors? Yeah? No, no, no, no, no! Don't go looking at your groin again. It's cerebral—it's cognition. That's right; it's the brain. Thirty-five percent of the receptors involve the brain and cognition. So say I have a patient named Ralph who is the vice president of Greengrass Bank (I hope there is no real person like that; but trust me, I have many who fit this category). He'll come to me as a patient, and I'll ask a few social questions. "Where do you work, Ralph?" "Oh down on um, um, you know—the street that goes by the delicatessen? Um … Damn! I'm drawing a blank, but you know the one I mean." Yeah, I know the street you mean because I still have cognitive function that is firing on eight cylinders, thanks to a symphony approach to my health and testosterone. Now don't get me wrong—I still have to work at it, but it truly is amazing to me the degree of cognitive delay with executives over the age of 45.

Okay, here comes the whopper! Five percent of testosterone works extraordinarily well to keep muscle tone, decrease subcutaneous fat, increase libido and sexual performance, and most importantly, help reduce abdominal fat. That's the fat that lies underneath the skin and the muscles and overlies the intestines—the previously mentioned omentum (apron cover). So that 5 percent is critically important; and so far, testosterone is the best medicine I've found for it since I started taking it in 1994 for heart protection.

Now you may be asking yourself why your testosterone is low. Was it all from the genes of your family's black sheep Great-Uncle Ralph? Calm down, big boy. You're still a stud. It's just that as we age (excuse me, mature), our hormones decrease rapidly. This usually occurs at age 40 to 45—just about the same time as menopause in women. By the way, this loss of testosterone also occurs dramatically in women, and it is seldom addressed or treated by physicians. Now here comes a big apology. A lot of physicians are only now catching on to this. Why? Because their patients have caught on to it. The patient approaches his physician and says that he had his testosterone tested at one of the local pharmacies; and lo and behold, it's on the low side. The physician may answer with one of two responses. He may say that the level is still within the normal range, although low. That, from my standpoint, is an inappropriate answer. You want your hormones to be in the 30 to 35 year old range. The second answer is just as debilitating. He may say, "Testosterone is low, so let's raise it up." That's the way we were taught to handle low levels of anything, and I do apologize. Unfortunately with hormones, that's not the way it works. When prescribing or taking testosterone, one must know that testosterone converts to estrogen. Estrogen is a hormone (yes, guys, you've got it, and lots of it as you get older!), and estrogen creates fat. The fat that it creates usually goes to the omentum or intra-abdominal fat. Now here's the problem: The intra-abdominal fat from the omentum actually is a living organ; and as a living organ, it makes a product. What do you think that product is? Bingo. You get to go on Jeopardy. It makes estrogen.

That estrogen then makes more fat, and that fat makes more estrogen, which makes more fat. I guess that's enough because I'm sure you get the picture. So giving you testosterone is going to give you a little more libido; it will give you a little more strength during your workouts. But it will also increase your abdominal girth almost assuredly unless the estrogen is blocked. Testosterone can also be transformed into another hormone called dihydro-testosterone. That's the one that helps make you bald and can enlarge your prostate a smidge. You need to block that as well. So you can see that it's not just as simple as "give me some testosterone." That won't fix it. The question is how do we balance all of these hormones?

Please know that testosterone does not cause prostate cancer—period. I'm sorry that so many doctors think otherwise. The facts are indisputable. However, one caution: if you have cancer, adding testosterone could theoretically encourage its growth. We never prescribe testosterone for men or women undergoing cancer therapy.

The important factor to realize with testosterone, as with all of your hormones, is that after age 40 or 45, it decreases. Please look at the graph below, and you'll see that at 30, your hormones are up in the upper left hand corner, but see how it swoops down? By the time you're in your 60s and until you die, your hormones decrease dramatically. What's the problem with that? Unfortunately, as hormones decrease, you increase your weight, which increases the propensity for hypertension, which increases the risk of coronary artery disease, which increases the risk of stroke, which increases your risk for diabetes, etc. Hormone balancing and taking a healthy lifestyle step in the right direction is the single most important thing that you can do—and do it now!

Along with estrogen, another prominent hormone that plays a role in men's health is progesterone. It's a very calming hormone—one

Hormones versus Age

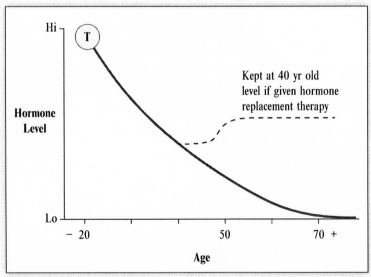

that enhances cognition just like testosterone. It can also lower estrogen, which is an inflaming hormone related to certain cancers, such as breast cancer in women and prostate cancer in men. Yep, progesterone lowers estrogen! How cool is that? Progesterone can be given as a topical cream with properties identical to your natural hormones.

And then there's cortisol. Cortisol is a hormonal substance created by the adrenal glands, which are little fellows that sit on top of your kidneys. They create a number of other substances, but cortisol is one of the more important ones. Think of cortisol as an energy hormone. When it's low, your energy will be extraordinarily low. When it's high, you may have more energy and more agitation; but unfortunately, it also tends to increase sugar and increase epinephrine, which increases insulin, which increase estrogen, which makes more fat and—oh yeah, there we go again—that big cycle. Are you starting to see how all of these hormones are connected? It really is a symphony, and just adding or subtracting a violinist is not the answer! By the way, the conductor with the baton is *you*—not your physician. Think of your physician as the instrument tuner.

Insulin is perhaps the most important instrument in this symphony. Most people think of it as something that diabetics need to lower their sugar. The truth is that we all need it, and we all need it balanced. Insulin absolutely enhances sugar going into fat cells. Yes; as I've pointed out, it makes us fat. The apology that I give to all diabetics is that very often some type II diabetics are put on insulin and told to diet or lose weight. We're giving you something to make you fat, but we're asking you to lose weight. Now don't misunderstand me; insulin is a wonderful product, especially for those without any insulin (type I) or for those who had a burnout of the beta cells of the pancreas that produce insulin (using supplemental insulin is critical). Their medical emphasis is to lower carbohydrate sugars dramatically and help transport sugar into muscle and fat cells.

As a type I diabetic using insulin (thank you so much, Agent Orange!), I am so thankful for insulin, but it wreaks hell on my weight. Carb counting is now just part of my life. As mentioned, insulin is an inflamer. It can inflame the walls of coronary arteries and increase inflammatory parts in entities such as rheumatoid arthritis, fibromyalgia, and a host of other diseases. What's the bottom line? Insulin needs to be low, low, low. It's one of those tests your physician should order, although most seldom do. An insulin high comes from increased sugar, which transforms into fat cells. Fat cells mean increased weight, which equals increased inflammation.

Now let's mention a little bit about a hormone talked about mostly in gyms—growth hormone. Growth hormone is considered the grandfather of all hormones. It has been studied in terms of longevity and in terms of increased endurance and strength. Unfortunately, there aren't a number of excellent studies showing its efficacy, but there are a number of studies that show its incredible costs. Growth hormones come as a daily injection and will run anywhere from $800 to $1,000 per month. Is it effective? I think so, but it must be utilized under the strict control of a physician. It will raise blood sugar, so diabetics would need to be monitored very closely. Is it worth the cost? Right now, the answer is no for me. Would it be beneficial in the future? Probably, but I'll start taking it when it's $1.25 per day and we have more evidence-based studies of it.

And now, here's a beauty—thyroid hormone. This gets a little complicated, but you're big folks, so I know you can handle this one. I do have to apologize because men have been somewhat neglected in this area of medical care. When we mention thyroid disease, almost exclusively, we as physicians think of women! Unfortunately, that's just not the truth. Men are just as susceptible to thyroid disease, and it is just as under-diagnosed as, and perhaps more so than, in women. Here's how it works. Your thyroid gland is in your neck, and it is monitored by a signal coming from your brain (TSH). This monitor sort of yells at the thyroid to make more; so if your TSH is high, it's yelling loudly, "Give me more thyroid!" When the TSH is low, it's in its soft whisper voice saying, "You don't have to make a whole lot more thyroid hormones because I have plenty." Get the picture? TSH acts as an opposite indicator and influencer of making thyroid hormones, but it has no other functional capacity in the body that we currently know of. Having been sent the signal (TSH), the thyroid responds by making T4 and T3 (thyroid hormones). Now it makes a ton of T4, and the T4 peripherally in the body (liver, kidneys, etc.) converts to T3. Why is that important? Although T4 is made in a 20-times larger package than T3, it by itself does practically nothing. It *must* convert to T3—the active powerhouse hormone. Interestingly, if you're diagnosed with low thyroid function, you are usually given a medication called "synthroid," which is T4. Well, that's nice; but remember that T4 does very little in the body. So what good does it do giving synthroid unless it can convert to T3? Now you get it—not much! So T4 converts to T3, and T3 is a dynamite regulator of just about damn near everything in your body. Cognition is improved; heart stability is improved; and weight is improved, Metabolism, GI tract motility, and balancing of sex hormones are increased as well.

The thyroid could be an entire chapter—a large one at that—but the important formula is that T4 gets converted to T3. For those scientists out there, it's done by an enzyme called 5 prime deiodinase. Now what do you think would happen if that enzyme were to diminish or dissipate, just like everything else does in our bodies as we age? Yep, your T4 can stay pretty much the same. Your TSH determines that everything is fine because it's being told by T4 that it's okay, but you have hypothyroidism. You're sluggish, cognition is down, libido is down, and weight is gained. You're not making T3 free.

So putting all this into a nutshell, please know that we as physicians have been trained to lower the labs that are high and raise the labs that are low. This is an outdated form of scientific evaluation, but it is still in practice. So as that practice relates to the thyroid gland, your most important lab would be a free T3, not just a T3, T4, or TSH. If the free T3 is low and/or you have symptoms of hypothyroidism, treatment should be initiated. Synthroid is T4; and if that little enzyme that we talked about (5-deiodinase) isn't working, you can take all the T4 in the world, but it's just not going to help. Adding Cytomel (T3) will make a world of difference. It's also important to remember that thyroid disease is a clinical diagnosis. Long before tests were available, a well-versed family physician would listen to the complaints of weight gain, lethargy, hair loss, constipation, change in menses, change in cognition, and depression, and he would notice the lateral third of the eyebrows' absence and a host of other signs and symptoms. This is hypothyroidism. It is critically important when one is diagnosed with this disease that the consideration for not just T4 (Synthroid) but also T3 (Cytomel) be incorporated if needed.

There is another consideration that should be taken in relationship to this entire symphony of hormones. I'm talking again about our orchestral conductors: neurotransmitters—those neuro- or brain-signaling substances that involve every aspect of living. When they are out of sync, a person may experience depression, hyperactivity, ADD, weight gain, craving for certain foods, inability to concentrate, inability to sleep, and more. As you can see, the list of lifestyle and living patterns is totally under the influence of neurotransmitters. The major ones that we'll be discussing in the upcoming chapter on neurotransmitters will be serotonin, dopamine, GABA, norepinephrine, and glutamate.

Neurotransmitters are critically important. If your dopamine levels are low, the ability to avoid having chocolate cake or a 3 Musketeers Bar is non-existent. It's as though you cannot avoid sugars. Entities such as Milky Way bars, soft drinks, caffeine in coffee, alcohol, nicotine, and a host of others raise dopamine levels momentarily. Lo and behold, the sun rises, and we feel good again. Unfortunately, that only lasts about one hour. Then comes the crash and the repeated acts of cravings and consuming sugar as we need more and more carbohydrates/sugars or other dopamine-raising substances to feel awake.

A few supplements have been clearly related to the increased ability of our brains to think better, be calm, and decrease our cravings.

They are as follows: omega-3, CoQ10, a multivitamin (maybe), melatonin, arginine, acetyl L-carnitine, carnosine, d-ribose, nitric oxide, chromium, and water. Water—that's the most important one. What about cholesterol for the brain? Low cholesterol impairs all of our brain functions and thus causes the cognitive delay and confusion that patients on statins (cholesterol-lowering meds) complain about.

There are some supplements that we want to try to avoid as men over the age of 45, and those are calcium and iron. Studies have shown that these are toxic to our hearts and brains. Some men have a plethora of iron (ferritin), which can be evaluated with labs. Those patients are at higher risks for stroke and thrombosis (clots). The disease process is known as hemochromotosis, and it can have a familial pattern to it. The best treatment for this is donating blood.

I think the best caveat that can be given in terms of hormonal balancing is that it needs to be part of a symphony, and you must be evaluated and treated by a qualified MD. For references, consult The Institute of Functional Medicine (www.functionalmedicine.org), World Health Net (www.worldhealth.net), or the American Academy of Anti-Aging Medicine (www.a4m.com). In general, most family physicians and internists are not trained in orchestrating the symphony of these hormones. Sorry. Here's one last warning for those of us of the male persuasion. When you read this list of hormones and supplements, it reads something like this: "Blah, blah, blah, blah ... testosterone!" By the way, if you have your testosterone tested, order the free testosterone as well as the total testosterone. The free testosterone usually accounts for your symptoms. You can actually have a normal total testosterone level while also having a sub-optimal free testosterone level. You could benefit from testosterone, in that case, depending upon your symptoms. One caveat: testosterone, when prescribed, can convert to estrogen if given in high doses. Estrogen makes fat; so with high doses of testosterone: "Hello, beer belly." There are substances (for example: zinc) and prescription medications (anastrazole) that prevent that conversion to estrogen. I hope that the description above shows how important testosterone is while also emphasizing the importance of all of the other hormones. They really do need to be part of a symphonic approach for you holistically. Balance them all, and yes, your "boys" will be happy again.

CHAPTER 10

Female Hormones

"This one's too hot; this one's too cold.
Mmmmmm...this one's just right."
—Goldilocks

I have yet to come across a woman who doesn't seem to understand hormones innately. I really applaud you, and I wish I could bottle your acceptance of them and take it to every male so that they could take a sip. If you skipped the last chapter on male hormones, go back and read the beginning of it. I know you may not be a man, but it's relevant—I promise. Read until you hit the end of the information about testosterone. The first part of the chapter—on balancing hormones and healthcare—is significant to you. The importance of knowing the information on testosterone will make more sense later in the chapter.

For women, perhaps one of the most important hormones to look at first and foremost is insulin. I touched upon this in the male section, and it applies here as well. It's really a very basic formula and comes down to this: what we take in for food has an effect. It's just that simple. So if you eat protein or fat, you will get practically no response from insulin. Protein does indeed raise insulin, but minimally. (Protein can convert to sugar.) What does raise insulin? You got it, kiddo—sugar. Most particularly, I'm talking about processed sugar in foods such as cakes, candies, and those delicious brownies that you make at Christmas. But as I mentioned earlier, some of the other sugars that we take in—and take in to excess—are through eating fruits and starches.

Of course, some are not as highly sugared as others. Bananas are through the roof and so are watermelons. Any berry, however, is low on the glycemic (or sugar intake) index. So blueberries and blackberries are always appropriate. Please take this to heart: there ain't no such thing as a free lunch. Sorry for the pun, but I mean this: yes, strawberries have a lower sugar content than some other fruits, but a bowl of strawberries is still a ton of sugar. A bowl of blueberries is still a ton of sugar. A baked potato is also sugar. What's a carbohydrate (think of it as the same as a sugar) that you would never think of as raising your blood sugar? You might answer broccoli or asparagus. Everybody thinks of those as amazingly healthy—and indeed they are because they have high fiber content. However, they still have sugar; and for diabetics, the quantity has to be monitored.

Why all this hoopla about carbohydrates? Again, to be repetitive, there are no bad foods. There's just too much of them. The higher the sugar content, the greater the inflammation it will cause systemically. How does all this work? It's pretty simple (at least for you women. Lord, help me with the men!). The contents of a high-sugar diet raise your insulin level. They also raise your estrogen level. When insulin is raised, your body closes down your fat cells and will not allow the energy or food that's stored there to come out and be utilized. Thus, you continue to grow larger and larger fat cells.

Now here is the tricky part. As your estrogen increases, it creates more fat, and fat creates more estrogen. I have lots of women coming to me saying they're menopausal, their estrogen is low, and they can't lose weight. I say to them that their estrogen is actually too high. It goes against everything they've ever read or heard; but remember, there are many types of estrogen. The estrogens that create more fat, particularly in the abdomen (omentum), are those that are increased when one ingests sugar. (Of course, estrogen will also go up if you're taking the craziest of the crazy medications for hot flashes: Premarin.) So when you consume sugar, estrogen and insulin go up. They both increase fat, and they both prevent energy that has been stored in fat cells from coming out. Unfortunately, they also open up the door to allow more sugars to be transported as triglycerides into the fat cells.

So back to my patients—after these women tell me that they can't lose weight and I tell them that their estrogen is elevated, they will immediately say, "You've got to be a quack. I've had a hysterectomy, my uterus is out, my ovaries are out, and my vagina is out! There is nothing down there but a pair of legs." Well, let's check. And of course, her labs show that her estrogen is elevated. How can that be?

When we look at the labs, they show increased sugar. We find that they are experiencing just what I've already explained: as they eat carbohydrates and sugars, their insulin increases and so does their estrogen. The increase in estrogen and insulin leads to that vicious cycle in which estrogen and insulin make fat, and that is a no-win situation. If one has a depletion of a neurotransmitter such as dopamine, it is almost impossible for that patient to beat their cravings, and they will gain weight.

So it really does come down to basics: if you want to maintain homeostasis (stability in the body metabolically) in relation to your insulin, you must concentrate on proteins, fats, and high-fiber carbohydrates for consumption—not sugars. (Vegetables with high fiber will usually be dark green.) Keeping your fruits and vegetables under 80 grams of carbohydrates total per day is ideal. As mentioned, for an easily downloaded version of the glycemic index, go to www.glycemicindex.com. Concentrate on items below 60 on the scale.

So to those women who come into my office with high estrogen, I would explain that they can be eating pansies and pebbles, and it really will not matter in this vicious cycle of insulin and estrogen producing fat and then fat producing more estrogen unless there is balance. Add a smidgen of exercise after balancing hormones and intake amount, and you have a painless weight loss program. By the way, I really do mean a painless program, especially the exercise. If you are running 3 miles a day, in my opinion, you are just beating yourself up. Now if that is your thing, please feel free. But for most of us, as I discussed in the chapter on activities, resistance training with bands, weights, or body resistance exercises (including yoga) and 10 minutes of any type of activity program are all that's needed to lower insulin. These activities can be walking, gardening, rowing, exercising on using an elliptical. (My favorite is walking for 30 minutes.) If you do 5 to 10 minutes of resistance training before each meal, you'll not only decrease your food craving, but you'll also lower the insulin surge that comes with every meal.

Now back to the topic of estrogen. Let's talk about those hot flashes. Whew. ... ain't they something! No man will ever understand them, so don't even try to explain them. If you really want to have some fun, give your husband 1,000 milligrams of niacin—yep, the vitamin—and he will experience that wonderful feeling of being on fire from the inside out for about 30 minutes to an hour! Having said that, what treatments are available for you? At the present, hopefully, nobody is using Premarin. You know the old story that Premarin stands for: **pre**gnant **mar**e ur**ine**. That's right; pregnant horses are stalled and catheterized for urine, and the product Premarin is manufactured from the extract. There is nothing in Premarin that is natural to your body.

There are today, however, bioidentical hormones that are chemically identical to the hormones that are in your body. These are manufactured from yams and soy. Using a product that would include hormones such as estriol, estradiol, and progesterones at night will alleviate the symptoms of hot flashes dramatically. There may be a difficulty in patients who have had prior cancer, particularly breast cancer; their physicians loathe promoting these hormones. There is no way around that at the present time other than to make your own decision on the efficacy of it. Many patients wait 5 years without recurrences of their cancer before using bioidentical hormones.

Currently, there are also many natural products to help relieve the symptoms of hot flashes and bed soakings. I think the major point is to realize that these issues are not minimal complaints. These are absolutely, positively debilitating and can currently be alleviated in nothing flat. And no, antidepressants are not the only answer. Some natural products available to relieve menopausal symptoms are black cohosh, evening primrose, and ashwaganda, to name a few.

For your overall health, you must also look at your progesterone levels. Progesterone is a hormone that is manufactured in your body as well. It is actually made from cholesterol, as are all of the female hormones. Progesterone is the absolute antithesis of estrogen. It is a non-inflammatory hormone and helps with weight loss and sleep. There are many studies that indicate that progesterone has an anti-cancer effect as well. Progesterone can be made from yams but is not the same as progestin. Progestin is made commercially, much like Premarin, in the form of medications such as Provera. The progesterone can be taken orally or topically as a cream. I prefer topically as a cream because the medication bypasses the liver, and I recommend as few medications going through the liver as possible. Overall, progesterone is deflaming throughout the body. It's the calming antithesis of inflammation. Estrogen, on the other hand, is totally inflaming (is there a man among us who isn't familiar with PMS?). It can also be related to cancer initiation.

And although most women wouldn't think about it, you also need to balance your testosterone. Wow! Most women are hypogonadal after the age of 40. That is just a big term that means "you ain't got no mojo," plain and simple. Testosterone is a valid entity, as mentioned in the male section, for heart protection and brain function/cognition protection, as well as for maintaining muscle tone, reducing subcutaneous fat, and, finally, increasing libido. Sixty percent of your testosterone goes to heart protection, 35% is for cognition and brain enhancing, and 5% is for loss of fat as well as increased libido and muscle tone. That's right, libido and loss of subcutaneous fat represents only 5%. Nonetheless, it is a powerful 5%. I don't believe I have tested a single woman over the age of 45 whose testosterone is normal. It is one of the most under-evaluated, under-treated and under-tested hormones for women over the age of 40. I'm sorry!

Testosterone can be given as a cream, and it is highly effective for women with vaginal dryness and even stress incontinence (spilling a little urine during the day with coughing or laughing). Stress incontinence can be treated with testosterone placed around the urethra (where the urine comes out). It works fabulously well. Now there is a tremendous set of symptoms that can be relieved by simply utilizing testosterone cream. Again, we will all lose our hormones. It's just a fact of nature. At 25, your hormones were raging, and you were necking in the back of a '76 Thunderbird. Now, at 45, it's vaginal dryness, lack of libido, and decreased cognition and drive. There's that overwhelming feeling that echoes, "Is there any end to this blah state I'm in?" I would hasten to say that low testosterone is at least 60% of the reason for those symptoms.

When you have labs drawn for testosterone, be sure that it is the free-testosterone form that you are looking for. Most physicians, if asked, will order for serum testosterone. That testosterone is bound to a protein and is essentially ineffective. Free testosterone is the level that you want to test, and you want it at the level of a 30 to 35 year old. That's at least at 75% of the normal range. So if your normal scores are 1 to 10, you need to be at 7. Unfortunately, you really do need to be tested for this because, like I mentioned in the last chapter, testosterone can convert to estrogen; and estrogen, when not checked, can yield weight gain and other side effects. So get tested and take testosterone if you need it. And no, you're not going to grow Arnold Schwarzenegger muscles or a moustache.

Perhaps the biggest failure that we in the medical profession are culpable for is not evaluating the thyroid function appropriately. Again, we get lost in the mumbo jumbo of various tests, most of which are unnecessary. As I mentioned in the previous chapter, the thyroid makes T4 and T3. T4 gets converted to T3 by an enzyme (5'-deiodase); and although it is made at 20 times the volume of T3, T4 is minimally effective in terms of what thyroid hormone is meant to do. T3, on the other hand, is extremely potent for increasing metabolism, preventing hair loss, and increasing cognition, heart protection, energy, and weight loss. So, if your free T3 is low, then taking T4 isn't necessarily going to help you much unless the converting enzyme (5'-deiodinase) is maximally functioning. If the enzyme isn't working, the lab that your physician normally obtains (T4) will be normal, but your T3 (not normally tested) will be low. On paper, you will look thyroid normal, but clinically, you'll be too pooped to pop.

T3 can be taken as a separate medication (Cytomel) or in combination with T4 from a compounding pharmacy or as a combination of thyroid extract. It's keeping thyroid at that 30 to 35-year-old range that is important. If normal in your doctor's lab is 2 to 10, you need to be at 6 to 8. Just because you are at 3 or 4 does not make you at a normal level (maybe normal for an untreated 90 year old).

These lab values, of course, must be taken into consideration with your symptoms. Do you have the symptoms of hypothyroidism? Then I don't even really care what your lab value is. You have hypothyroidism. Let's treat you at a minimal dose and see how you do. I have yet to have a patient come back and say, "This stuff stinks." They love it. And if you are on thyroid medication at the present time, it may be that the Synthroid, which is T4, is not being converted to T3. You may need supplementation with T3 instead.

Here's another thought: you may indeed have your thyroid function affected because of medications or low supplements. If you are low in zinc, iodine, magnesium, or B vitamins, you're going to have a difficult time converting T4 to T3. What about medications? Are you on an antidepressant or a beta blocker? These and others will dramatically affect your thyroid function.

I have one last point of interest before leaving the hormones, and that is the fact that when we speak of estrogen, we are really talking about a variety of estrogen. The major ones that are looked at particularly in the arena of cancer are 2 hydroxy, 4 hydroxy, and 16 hydroxy estrogens. The 2 hydroxy estrogen is extremely effective in terms of fighting cancer, keeping brain mentation, and staying heart healthy. We like that stuff, but 4 hydroxy and 16 hydroxy are related to inflammation. Yep, that's right—inflammation in all forms. Inflammation in terms of cancer, inflammation in terms of fibromyalgia, and inflammation in terms of arthritis and in a host of others. So what's the goal? Let's keep the 4 and 16 hydroxys down.

At the present time, there are a number of medical ways to keep those down; however, they are utilized primarily for cancer patients. There is a natural supplement called Dim, or chemically, Indole 3 Carbinol. It has been shown to enhance estrogen breakdown toward the 2 hydroxy paths, avoiding creation of 4 and 16 hydroxy. This supplement has absolutely no side effects, and it really comes from cruciferous vegetables. Is there any reason not to take Dim? You tell me because I can't think of one. Again, this supplement can be obtained from any one of a variety of vendors in the appendix.

I would be remiss if I didn't mention that menopause in general is a topic that involves all of these hormonal entities in truly symphonic chaos. Talk about cacophony! But it doesn't take much to stabilize and relieve symptoms. It does, however, take a lot of caring, and I apologize for the fact that most of us as male physicians tend to slight this. It is absolutely a hormonal dysfunction. The key point to remember is that all of it can be managed. It does take caring, and it does take an understanding of neurotransmitters as well. We will talk about neurotransmitters in the next chapter, but please realize how your neurotransmitters, dopamine, GABA, serotonin, norepinephrine, and glutamate, along with others, really do need to be balanced to help with menopause. It's only with balanced neurotransmitters that we can keep our head on course. Also know that all of the symptoms of menopause vary from patient to patient. You may have a friend (but probably not for long) who never experiences so much as a bead of sweat during menopause. Women like this should be banned to a desert island. However, the majority of women will experience all variations; and the major takeaway point is that it is an everyday annoyance that will affect your personalities, drives, initiatives, libido, and living experience unless it is managed appropriately.

So find a physician who cares and is trained in this field. You're way more than worth it, as the hair commercial claims, and balancing your neurotransmitters will certainly help.

CHAPTER 11

Neurotransmitters

*"Have patience. All things are difficult
before they become easy."*—Saadi

I really like my car. The seats, the radio, and the air conditioner are great, but the engine gets practically no attention from me whatsoever—yet it is the core of my car. When I get on an airplane, I love the wings and the little bags of peanuts, but I don't get to see much of the person who really runs the show—the pilot. And what about surgery? If you've ever had any surgery, you might spend some time talking to the surgeon, but the person you won't spend much time with is the anesthesiologist. He really is the one running the show. When I had my heart surgery, a plumber could have moved around the tubes in my heart—a very well-trained plumber, that is. However, for the anesthesiologist to put me to sleep, to bring me that close to death, and to bring me back again, well, that's a true skill. So my point is that the seldom-seen, the seldom-discussed, and the seldom-thought-about things in life are often times the most critically needed aspect of living well. And this brings us to neurotransmitters.

What the heck are neurotransmitters? Well, we've mentioned them a number of times, but now let's get into a little more detail. One of the definitions we can use is that they are the hormones of the brain. They are the messengers of neurological information from one cell to another, and they are the essence of all of our lifestyle activities—both physical and mental. So whether the topic is depression or craving food or lack of libido or whatever, neurotransmitters are involved, and they must be coordinated and stabilized. Here comes my biggest apology of all: We as physicians just don't know how to stabilize neurotransmitters because we haven't been taught. The treatment and evaluations are leading edge. They are really the forefront of a symphonic approach to managing the entire body, and we're just beginning to realize the complexity!

There is now testing available to determine your neurotransmitter levels. This testing can be done through a variety of different companies, one of which is Life Extension (www.lef.org). You can even order this testing yourself. In general, it involves a saliva test and a urine sample. Measurements of your neurotransmitters will be sent to you. One of the companies, Senesco (www.senesco.com), will even tell you what products can enhance the neurotransmitters that you are particularly deficient in.

A few of the neurotransmitters that are major players in your health and wellness are serotonin, dopamine, GABA, glutamate (a measure of inflammation), and norepinephrine/acetocholine.

If your serotonin level is low, you are going to feel depressed and have decreased energy levels. Your mental activity will be impaired as well, and you'll be living in the land of the "blahs." GABA is the cousin of serotonin and causes similar feelings. What about dopamine? When that is low, you will experience a decrease in pleasure and an increase in weight and food craving. Your libido will decrease as well. Multi-tasking will be out of the question. You may also sense an increased need for sleep. That is your body's first aid for trying to rebuild the dopamine levels.

Norepinephrine is really your lighter fluid. When everything else is down, norepinephrine, or adrenaline, will keep you going. Well, norepinephrine and adrenaline are fine for running from a tiger, but using them to get to work will increase your heart rate, your blood pressure, as well as inflammation. Again, that's all terrific when you're desperately fleeing for your life, but norepinephrine is not for everyday use.

Probably one of the best and easiest to read texts on neurotransmitters is by Dr. Eric Braverman. His book *The Edge* is undeniably accurate and understandable. If the word neurotransmitter is new to you, or if you think that the word serotonin only relates to using an antidepressant, it would be well worth your while to read *The Edge*.

Unfortunately, in today's society, this is exactly what most of us think: "My serotonin level is low, and my serotonin is related to depression." Or we think, "I'm depressed so I need an antidepressant." I'm here to tell you that is just *not* the case. It is not that antidepressants aren't worthwhile in certain patients; but they are, in my opinion, one of the most over-prescribed medications in the United States (probably right up there with statins!). What's the deal? The simple pathway for most of us runs like this: We have stressors in our life, and the stressors aren't simply our spouse, our children, our bills, or our job. Sure, those are extremely important, so let's classify those as emotional. Along with emotional stressors, there are other stressors that I've mentioned including tobacco, caffeine, alcohol, exercise, and—most importantly—sugar. There are a host of others, but these take the Oscar.

With these stressors in our bodies, we produce multiple free radicals (or little BBs) that beat up everything inside. Most particularly, they beat up the lining of our arteries. The other thing they do, of course, is deplete the elements that make serotonin and dopamine, our neurotransmitters. We often don't usually take in enough of the nutrients that are required to make neurotransmitters. So if you want to increase your serotonin or dopamine levels, you should increase your phenylalanine, your tryptophan, and your 5HTP. You should increase your leucine and isoleucine and increase your B vitamin intake. Use C vitamins as well.

That's a very simple version of how to increase your serotonin or dopamine levels. It's not as if you can put all of those substances into a cup of hot water, stir them around, and BOOM—you're fixed! However, this version does mean that there are supplements, including all of those, which increase our neurotransmitters. Notice that antidepressants were not on that list. The side effects from antidepressants alone are enormous—weight gain, lethargy, dry mouth, interactions with other medications, loss of libido, etc.

Having harmoniously balanced neurotransmitter machinery allows us to focus and discern. In this day and age, a lot of people have lost those abilities. We are constantly inundated with concepts like health, wellness, love, medicine, and intelligence—but what do they actually mean? Are we able to discern the truth? Not without an intact neurotransmitter cognition factory. When I have asked a patient what a good wellness program would be for him or her, my question is always the same: "What is wellness to you?" Again, going back to my 96-year-old aunt-in-law, can we settle and agree on the fact that wellness is being "better today than yesterday." It has very little to do with what vitamins you're taking or what exercise you're doing. Is there sanity in your life? Are you able to focus and look outside yourself? Like I've said before, the fact is this: We are all going to die—it's just a question of how. Sorry.

CHAPTER 12

Supper Mints

"If someone offers you a breath mint,
accept it."—H. Jackson Brown, Jr.

*H*ave you ever been to one of those really fancy restaurants? You know the kind—they have tons of food, linen napkins without stains (unlike those in my house), and creamy desserts—don't forget the lavish bill as you leave. To make the bill more palatable, there's a nice peppermint at the register—at no charge. Why a peppermint? What's wrong with caramel? Well, here's the secret: As you were eating, you were also swallowing air and becoming very bloated. Peppermint has an amazing ability to relax the valve in your esophagus (your food pipe), so out comes the bloat or air. Ahh, the relief. The discomfort subsides, and you might be tempted to think, "I could have handled one more piece of the lemon meringue pie!" And that's why peppermint candies have been given after dinner for decades. By the way, coffee and tea (because of the caffeine) will do the same.

Now that little peppermint fact might seem like nothing more than trivia for a contestant on Jeopardy, but here's my point: Peppermint works and is very helpful. But if you take it daily or in excess, you'll spend the rest of your life urinating. Yup, it makes you pee! Good stuff, but it has its side effects. What a nice segue into supplements.

Supplements have become a booming business today. Some of them actually work and are helpful. However, the other side of that coin is that some are shams and can have terrible side effects—particularly by interacting with prescription medications.

Obviously I can't cover every supplement, but I can give you some tips and resources on some of them. My first advice is to see a trained physician or health provider who is well-versed in supplements and vitamins. Use the products those physicians have or offer, as they will carry the best and safest products. Please use the websites listed in the back of the book as examples of reputable suppliers. You can learn a tremendous amount about vitamins and supplements from a great book: *What You Must Know About Vitamins, Minerals, Herbs and More*. The author—Dr Pamela Smith, MD—is an esteemed clinician on healthy living and supplements.

So where should we begin? My guess is that the builders of the space shuttle had the same question; and like them, I'm a big believer in being safe. So let's start with the safe stuff—uh oh—there is no such thing as safe when it comes to supplements, herbs, or vitamins. The best we can hope for is "probably ok" and "might help." If you can live with that (pun intended), here are some pointers:

(If you're pregnant or on chemotherapy, disregard everything that follows; you're on restricted protocols. Don't take supplements without your physician's advice.)

Everyone has heard of Omega 3 fatty acids and fish oil (sometimes written as DHA/EPA). These are actually quite safe, but they can prolong bleeding. So if you're on a blood thinner, please take these with caution and ask for your physician's advice. Their properties are legendary, but you'd have to eat fish daily to reach a therapeutic level of Omega 3s without a supplement. Omega 3 helps with cognition, heart function, lowering lipids, and avoiding clots and arrhythmias. They also enhance insulin function and have a host of other positive results. All this and more can be yours for just the possibility of an occasional fishy burp. (Using Krill instead helps to eliminate the burp.) The only creatures that do not need to take fish oil are … fish!

Another favorite supplement of mine is CoQ10. It's a fat-soluble nutrient found in nuts, broccoli, salmon, spinach, and beef heart. (Mmm, nothing like a nice beef heart sandwich. Doesn't that sound tasty?!) Coenzyme Q 10 is made and functions in nearly every cell of your body. That fact itself wins CoQ10 the Oscar for supplements. However, it's also responsible for providing cellular energy. Have caution, though. Like Omega 3, CoQ10 can also increase bleeding and interact with other medicines. Once again, discuss this with your physician before taking the supplement. CoQ10 has been shown to be effective in fighting heart disease, diabetes, asthma, high blood pressure, and many other ailments. It also aids in weight loss.

Here's one of the recent headliners: D3. Now it sure looks like a vitamin—and indeed, it is a derivative of vitamin D—but it's actually a pro-hormone. It facilitates other hormones, strengthens bones, fights breast and prostate cancer, increases metabolism, and is used effectively in weight loss protocols. It's a fat-soluble substance, so it's best absorbed when eating a fatty meal or before sleep because of its calming response. D is dynamite.

Vitamin B is really 11 entities. (For the super-curious, they are B1 [thiamine], B2 [riboflavin], B3 [niacin], B5 [pantothenic acid], B6 [pyridoxine], B7 [biotin], B9 [folate], B10 [para-aminobenzoic acid], and B12 [cobalamin, choline, inositol].) They are collectively the B complex and are best taken as a group or complex. Now I know that B12 gets the spotlight in most offices and articles, but each one of the Bs plays a critical part in over 300 chemical bodily reactions. I never miss a day. The same is true for vitamin C, which is a fabulous anti-oxidant. Thank you, Linus Pauling.

The next substance I want to mention is not a supplement per se, but I never miss a night of taking the element Magnesium. Five hundred mgs at bedtime is a fantastic aid to sleeping. Not enough reason for you to use it? It acts as an amazing muscle relaxant, stool softener, migraine preventive, insulin enhancer, and cardiac arrhythmia protectant. Magnesium—not just a flash in the pan! (Sorry, a pun for chemistry buffs.)

This supplements chat is clearly minimal and is in no way meant to endorse them. They are, for the most part, safe and efficacious; but the list of supplements and vitamins is close to endless. Some substances can be dangerous, as innocuous as they sound, such as multivitamins with Iron. Iron can cause GI bleeding and can be very toxic to the heart, liver, and kidneys. Please always remember Schneider's rule: The difference between supplements, medicines, vitamins, and poison is the dose. Now remember rule number 2: If you don't need it, don't take it. There are laboratory tests that can determine your personal levels and needs for supplements and vitamins. Grab the facts and leave the opinions to the politicians.

CHAPTER 13

Grandma Stuff

"If God had intended us to follow recipes,
he wouldn't have given us grandmothers."
—Linda Henley

Who doesn't remember Grandma and her wisdom? A lot of my early health instruction came from my grandma. If you can't remember your grandma, it must have been your mother or some wise sage. Either way, they always had disciplined comments for us. Remember? Eat all of your vegetables; don't sit close to the television; don't put anything in your ear smaller than your elbow. I thought I'd mention just a few of those comments that actually have a basis in science. This advice came naturally to Grandma, and they go something like this:

Posture Grandma was always telling me to stand up straight. Yes, posture actually is important. It says who you are, and thus, it tells *you* who you are. Standing up straight tells you and the world that you face life straight up. It also improves your breathing. It decreases the incidence of osteoporosis and curvature of the spine. How can you tell if you're doing it correctly? Well, once or twice a day, back yourself against a wall. Have your heels, your buttocks, your shoulders, and your head touch the wall. Pull your shoulders back, and that's straight posture. No, you can't keep that up throughout the day. You will start to slump, and that's what you want to try to work against. So practicing proper posture a couple of times a day, by backing yourself against a wall, is a nice reminder that posture is important. So go ahead; hit the wall.

Breathing   When I was hurt and crying, or when I was scared in the dark, my grandma would hug me and say, "Just be calm and breathe." Breathing is a form of oxygenation, increasing cognition and relaxation. If you're anxious before a presentation, practice ten of these breaths: Inhale to the count of six and then exhale slowly while counting to six again—maybe eight if you can do it. You will be amazed at how it calms you down. Breathing is, without a doubt, the most critical aspect of our life. It is our core, and it is our essence. But do we inhale correctly? Not a chance. What is the proper technique? Well, to practice it, lie on the floor and put your hand on your abdomen. Take a deep breath in and watch your abdomen rise. It is your abdomen rising toward the ceiling that you want to experience. When you exhale properly, you should feel your abdomen retracting toward your backbone. Inhale, exhale; using this format will establish muscle memory, and you will develop a pattern of proper breathing and oxygenation.

Meditation   Now Grandma probably never mentioned meditation because she may have never heard of the word. What she probably did do was tell you to pray or to sit in the corner when you were bad. Well, I'm not going to tell you either of those, but I will tell you to meditate—to sit quietly in the corner (or any quiet place you choose) at least once a day. It doesn't have to be 30 minutes of Zen "ohms" during which you try to eradicate your mind to the point of nothingness. Leave that to the Buddhist monks. But for you and me, take 5 minutes—yep, that's right, only 5 minutes—to sit quietly. You can meditate after lunch or when you wake up or before bed. It doesn't matter when. When meditating, your mind will try to bring in any piece of news or information it can to interrupt. Don't try to fight that. It's nearly impossible; there's no way I can clear my mind. (That's surprising because there is very little of my mind left.) So when extraneous thoughts flood my mind in meditation, I don't fight them. I don't get angry or consider myself a loser guru. I simply focus my attention on the air passing through my nostrils. Can meditation really help? There is a philosophical aphorism that says it all: "Look within—the secret is inside of you." (Hui Neng)

The secret here is to simply concentrate on the breath. Sit with your mouth closed and feel the air passing in and out through your nostrils. Sometimes, to avoid the thoughts that creep in while I meditate, I will use a mantra or word as I breathe in. As I inhale, I mentally say to myself "accept," and as I exhale, I mentally say "aware." "Accept" means to accept what's going on right now in every area of my life. "Aware" is a mental note for me to be aware of everything, such as my wife's look or my child's mood. Whatever it is, be aware.

Water   Yeah, how 'bout that wet stuff? Grandma always told me to drink 8 glasses of water a day. What's the science behind that? None—sorry. From a scientific standpoint, we don't have a clue how much water you should take in. The best answer is to keep your urine clear. Light is acceptable, but yellow or dark yellow is pure dehydration. So 8 or more glasses of fluids per day is acceptable. The importance of water is indescribable. Water is key. Essentially, we are an ocean, and we need to refill that ocean as we deplete water every day.

Teeth I remember my grandma's teeth. They sat in a glass at night, and Grandma warned me that mine would be there as well unless I took care of them. Whenever someone is talking about "wellness"—whatever that is—one of the most forgotten aspects of it is one's teeth. But teeth are critically important to your wellness. Did you know that the reason that lions, the kings of the jungle, die is that they only eat raw meat and get no calcium from the bones that they gnaw on? They lose their teeth and die of starvation. Holy mackerel—the king of beasts dies because of poor dentition. How bad is that?

So, absolutely get dental checks twice a year. Dental cleanings? Absolutely. What about that action that we hate so much—flossing? It turns out that flossing at least once a day is critically important to healthy gums. Poor dentition, including gums, has been related to cardiovascular disease, so I am a big believer in non-alcoholic mouthwash, brushings with the softest toothbrush available, and gum care by flossing. Here's a little tip: The only amount of toothpaste that you need is about the size of a pea. So put a pea-size amount on the end of your toothbrush and have at it. There, I've saved you at least 50% on toothpaste costs. Buy some floss with your savings.

Feet It didn't matter what kind of shoes I wanted—Grandma wanted them to fit and give support. She wouldn't buy me cool, high-top sneakers, so I had to have brown, properly fitting Oxfords. Ever play basketball in brown Oxfords? Feet are one of the more neglected entities in wellness healthcare. Diabetics particularly need to be aware that an infection, a bunion, or an ingrown toenail could lead to the loss of a foot. Yep—we're not playing around here, folks. You need to take care of your feet. Get the widest shoe you can. I think it's absolutely insane that we have women stuff their feet into these pointed, high-heeled, angled shoes. I mean, come on, it's 2013; let's get over that.

Ingrown toenails can be self-medicated by cutting a "V" in the center of the nail, and that occasionally works. Sometimes, placing a small wisp of cotton under the side of the ingrown nail will help as well. Don't hesitate to see a podiatrist, as podiatrists really are the wizards of feet. In general, the best thing to do for your feet is a shoe fitting. I don't care if you buy ten pairs of shoes a year if you can afford it, but get shoes that fit and are wide. When you buy a shoe, even if it's a running shoe, you should have at least a distance of your thumb's width between your big toe and the end tip of the shoe. I use two fingers, but then again, I'm diabetic.

Ears Remember when Grandma told you to turn down the radio? Well, she was right. Loud noises do indeed affect hearing. You can develop tinnitus, which is a big word we doctors like to throw around to confuse everybody. It simply means a constant noise in the ear. The most common cause for tinnitus is exposure to loud noise. As a former fighter pilot, I have it in both of my ears, and it's not going away. The best way to avoid it is to avoid loud noises when you are young. If the noise in your ear is unilateral, then you should seriously get it looked at. There are small tumors called acoustic neuromos, and they can present with the symptom of noise.

Eyes Like the young lad in the movie *A Christmas Story*, I always wanted a BB gun, but nooo—not from my grandma. She was convinced I'd shoot my eye out. Well, I never shot my eye out, but there are a lot more common diseases of the eye than BBs. What can I say? Once a year, it truly is worth having an ophthalmologist just look into the back part of your eye. That's when she or he dilates your eye and uses a scope for looking at the retina on the inside. This area has visible vessels, arteries, and veins. An astute physician can see plaque as showing atherosclerotic disease and can see what's called AV nicking, which is prominent in hypertension. Even tumors can be identified in the retina.

Skin   Skin is the largest organ in the body. Yep, it is an organ. Skin is a good indicator of how hydrated we are. (Thanks again for pushing water, Grandma.) Dry skin is an indicator of a chronic need for more hydration. Additionally, our skin shows little rascals such as moles and malignant tumors. Some of those rascals like basal cell carcinoma are easily eradicated. Basal cell carcinoma looks much like a doughnut; it will have a round ridge on the outside and a deep hole on the inside. You can also have, of course, squamous cell carcinoma. This is a bad actor and can spread. There are also various types of melanomas, but the best way to detect a melanoma is if it's multi-colored (i.e., bluish, purplish, reddish) with irregular margins. If in doubt, let the dermatologist check you out.

What about those sunburns? Clearly, sunburning is worse during mid-day, so if you're going to be out in the sun extensively and uncovered, then sun block is key, of course. The safest times to be in the sun are from 8:00 a.m. until about 10:00 a.m. and then around 4:00 p.m. until sundown. If you're a high-risk candidate for skin cancer (fair skin, red or blonde hair, blue eyes, and living in a region with high sun exposure) or have a family history of melanoma, a once-a-year, full-body evaluation by a dermatologist is well worth the investment and effort.

When you use sun block, remember that you are blocking the rays of the sun. The sun is a major source of vitamin D, which converts under the skin to vitamin D2 and then to the pre-hormone D3. D3 is one of the most salient pre-hormones, meaning it is currently being touted as a cognitive protector, cardiovascular protector, and breast cancer/prostate cancer preventative. D3 at 5,000 IU per day is a winner!

Mind   Of all the sage advice my grandmother gave me, none was more valuable than this: "As you think, so will you be." Among all the aspects of every physiologic and anatomical part of us as living beings, nothing defines us more as individuals than our functioning mind. Not having that brain functioning at full steam, without a doubt, is the most common deficiency of patients who come to see me for any variety of other ailments. Decreased cognition shows up in all types of symptoms including fatigue, lethargy, inability to concentrate, and easy forgetfulness. The mind is essentially a body part that follows the same axiom as everything else: use it or lose it. If you're not reading, learning to play an instrument, going online doing mental quizzes, or interacting, then do it!

Interactions with friends and neighbors are just as critically important to keeping your mind alive, well, and healthy as mental quizzes are. Interestingly, the Okinawans have the word *"moai."* A *moai* is a gathering at the end of the day by the Okinawans, who then commiserate, share in their day, and partake with their community. The Okinawan communities that follow this tradition have the highest number of centenarians on the planet. I think I may go next door and borrow a cup of sugar or ask what's cooking.

Sleep   "It's time for bed, no if's, and's, or but's." I think that's a direct quote from Grandma. Those are words of dread for every child and words of relief for every parent. The truth is that everybody wins with sleep. Sleep deprivation is one of the most prevalent and under-diagnosed disease entities in the United States. Yes, I said disease because, in fact, obstructive sleep apnea and inability to have full restful sleep is devastating. What will happen the following day after a poor night of sleep? An inability to concentrate, inability to focus, daytime fatigue, lack of energy, a host of other problems, and—here comes the

whopper—increased insulin. The increased insulin will increase
your cravings for food. You will gain weight. Your cortisol level
will also rise without adequate sleep and will initiate the onset
of diabetes. Additionally, remember that super-hormone called
growth hormone? The one that gives us strength and endurance
and is related to longevity? Well, guess what? Growth hormone
is produced and is maximally excreted while we sleep. It is produced throughout the day, but sleep is when it is at its premium.

Fun Stuff   Grandma always said, "Make today fun." I'm sure
you won't do all of these, but here are suggestions to make wellness fun, and I strongly recommend that you pick a few. When
you get bored with a couple, switch them out with some others.
These are not only healthy hints; they're a kick:

1. *Make lists.* Lists are great. Make a list of things that you
   want to do, things that are new and exciting, and things that
   are fun. Make a list with an exercise routine you're going to
   do, a new CD that you'd love to listen to, or a list of any and
   all projects for the day. Lists can be fun, especially the part
   where you cross items off.

2. *Take a walk.* Take it by yourself or with your family. This is
   a walk in addition to your activities and exercise. During the
   walk, concentrate on your breathing, much like the meditation that we talked about before. Look at the trees and see if
   you can find birds or ants climbing the bark. Sounds crazy,
   doesn't it? But honestly, focusing your mind on minutiae
   and on the beauty of nature will keep that mind alive.

3. *Walk as much as possible.* You know, the Japanese have a
   wonderful study that showed that diabetics who walked
   10,000 steps per day were able to come off their Type II insulin medications and most of their oral medications. I've got
   to tell you, I work out 7 days a week, and 10,000 steps is just

incredibly difficult. (It's roughly 4 miles.) I tell my patients to shoot for 1,000, then maybe 1,500, and then scoot it up to 2,500. Buying a pedometer to mark your progress is great. There's even an app for your phone that acts as a pedometer! (Now I'm just waiting for an app to think for me—no, I'm not!) Do a week at one level before you try to increase it by even 500 steps. That may be a little more sane for most people, including me.

4. *Have a half scoop of ice cream* if that's your thing. It is mine, and I truly love coffee ice cream. So Wednesday—hump day—I have half a scoop. I shouldn't; I'm diabetic. Wait a minute—who says I shouldn't? I can, and I love every bite of it.

5. *Make protein shakes.* Enjoying a protein shake for breakfast is a fabulous way to lose weight, and it will fill you for most of the morning. Start a weight-loss plan with a protein shake at least three times a week. Now what's the big deal about protein shakes? It has proteins, and it has fats. Remember that we want a shake that is very low in carbohydrates. Remember, carbohydrates up means insulin up. Insulin up means weight up. I know you get it. There are a number of protein shakes available; and just for reference, some of the best will have 1–3 of grams of carbohydrates, not the 15–18 grams in shakes that are sold commercially.

6. *Fast.* This is actually a fun one for the day. It means just consuming liquids. Now the liquids can include tomato juice, tea, coffee, water, or even water with Crystal Light— you decide. This is a fast from solid foods, and there are numerous studies which show the efficacy of fasting. I don't recommend this as a daily process; but once a month, it's actually very metabolically recharging. The fast is from

morning wake up until normal dinner at night. If you're diabetic, obviously watch your sugars as they may plummet. Fasts are not meant to be torture, just metabolism boosters.

7. *Die.* Now isn't that a weird recommendation for fun? But here's my point: Just as I mentioned before, pick a day, anytime of day. Lie down or do this when you first wake up. Feel your head, shoulders, buttocks, legs, and heels on the mattress. Breathe in, breathe out, and just remind yourself that this is the way you will lie one day for eternity. In yoga classes, we call it *shavasana*, and that is translated to mean "corpse pose." Why is that so important? Because we, as individuals, need to come to grips with our own death. I've mentioned this, but I can't say it enough: We should all have advance directives determining how we are going to die and what we want for ourselves in terms of medical care if no one is there to answer for us. Again, advance directives should be carried in your wallet or in your purse. Your family physician needs to know what your wishes are. It does no good to have this in your safe deposit box. Dying is an amazingly wonderful thing, and we need, as a people, to become more aware of its beauty.

8. *Give away five dollars.* How about giving $5.00 to the down and out? Not for gratification or a goody-two-shoes response from the down and out, but just give it freely. I usually say, "I think you dropped this," and I give it to them. I have never had anybody say, "No, it's not mine." It's always "Thank you" and "God bless." I'm not looking for God to bless me; I'm just looking to give someone who is down and out money that he or she can use. "But what if that person uses it for drugs, Doc?" I don't judge. I just give to someone in need. I leave the judging to the judges.

9. *Turn off the TV; turn off your cell phone, and turn off your computer.* It's absolutely amazing how your world will change for one day without any electronic devices. I know, all the people in business are sitting there saying they can't do it because they can't miss anything really important. Well, guess what? Today is your last day, and the likelihood of you dying tomorrow is just as real as you waking up and being alive. Nobody cares about your cell phone, your tweets, your twitters, or your e-mails. Just try it for a day—what can you lose? The world will not change. I think one of the greatest phrases of all times is this: "The sun will rise tomorrow without thy assistance." I like that.

10. *Don't talk.* This is a really tough one for most people because we want to be heard, we want to be listened to, and we want to feel important. Pick a day when you just don't talk—or when you do, it's really minimal. What's the point? The idea is to listen. Listen to the anxiety in those who are talking to you. Listen to the depression in those who are speaking to you. Listen to the needs and the joys of those who are talking to you. Listen; don't speak. There is a great aphorism that says, "If man can learn to sit in silence each day, there would be no need for war." I'm all about no war.

So you can see that none of this is genius work. It's just reiterating what you already know but, hopefully, reinforcing that the time to start doing this is *now*. Let's face it: life has gotten too complicated and too confusing with far too many stressors. Grandma, I can't accomplish all of the good things and the needed things that I should in every day, but I will make every day a little different. I will use some of your wisdom in each one of my days. Thanks, Grandma!

CHAPTER 14

Putting it All Together—The Humpty Dumpty Plan

"Poached, fried, or on the side."

You know, I hate to start a chapter with "I'm sorry," but I really am. You see, nobody really has it all together—particularly not me. What I *do* have is a game plan. This game plan has worked for me and gotten me through, over, and beyond more diseases than most physicians have seen in a lifetime. No, there isn't a guarantee that this will work for you—but it sure hasn't failed anyone in my practice, and it keeps me going day after day. So let's get started.

As I've mentioned a few times before, the first step is to find a wellness/innovative/out-of-the-box physician. There are a number of places you can go to find physicians like this, but it is most important that he or she be board-certified and extremely well-trained. A couple of good websites are www.a4m.com and www.functionalmedicine.org (The Institute of Functional Medicine). These are basically national clearinghouses for physicians who are interested in "wellness" alternative medicine. There are numerous excellent courses and even a certification and fellowship training. No, it's not recognized by the AMA, but I don't suspect that the AMA will certify any board certification in this field. The National Institutes of Health also has an excellent website: www.nih.gov. There are many other sources that list trained physicians, but the three above are my favorites.

What do you think is the best way to evaluate your current or future physician in terms of wellness, other than the criteria I've mentioned? I'll tell you what I do. I check my physician's demeanor, mind, and look. If my physician is 20 pounds overweight, has little personality, and isn't much into teaching, but is very much into having me run through nutritionists, nurse practitioners, exercise physiologists, machines, gadgets, and creams—then I'm sorry, but I'd look elsewhere. Using other healthcare practitioners is great, but your physician needs to be the one you spend most of your time with.

The physician who you see should also be ordering very specific labs. Your regular physician will order a blood count, a lipid panel, a fasting blood sugar, and a urinalysis. What you are looking for, however, is hormonal testing such as TSH, T4, and mandatorily a *free* T3. Remember that the free T3 is the test that truly determines the degree of your thyroid function. Testosterone is done similarly. Getting your serum testosterone is fine, but the real key is your free testosterone. The scores will vary greatly between men and women.

A serum insulin level and a hemoglobin A1C are dramatic markers not only for diabetes but also for the likelihood of developing diabetes. An hsCRP and arachidonic-to-EPA ratio are fabulous markers for inflammation within the body. Your physician should also measure your homocysteine level, which is specific for organ inflammation markers (intestines, liver, joints, uterus, ovary, etc). This physician should also measure hsCRP. That will indicate the inflammatory markers within the body and, most specifically, within the heart. On most lab scales, if it's severely above 3, then a cardiac workup is well-warranted. Be sure to ask your physician about all of these tests.

Other testing that is excellent and can be done from an office-based practice are ultrasounds to evaluate the carotid artery as well as the thyroid in the neck. This is a 30-second, painless procedure and gives an excellent indication of where you are now as a patient as well as where you are heading. In fact, numerous tests are available that are indicative of where your health is now and where your lifestyle is taking you. The levels for "normal" that I use for analyzing these tests may be far lower than what you or your physician are used to seeing. Let's say your fasting glucose is 115. A traditional diagnosis of diabetes would not take place until your blood sugar level is at least 126; but by the time your level is 126, your diabetes is well set in, and the damage is already accumulating its effects on your vessels. Thus, 99 is my top limit for a patient's fasting sugar; and certainly, I would encourage patients to be well under 90. It's a whole lot easier to avoid kayaking over a waterfall than to row back upstream.

Following the labs and special testing as warranted, a physical examination is obviously appropriate. We as patients consider a physician being hands-on as the gold standard when actually it is the least important aspect of the entire process. History—the information given to the physician in terms of symptoms, lifestyle, goals, etc.—is really the key to understanding the patient. Sure, it's great to listen to a patient's lungs on the physical exam; but if I want to know by your history that your symptoms might indicate lung cancer, I need to see your lung CT scan, plain and simple. My stethoscope can stay in my black bag.

Knowing a thorough history (including nutrition, exercise, stress evaluation, and sleep, etc.), physicals, labs, and a neurotransmitter profile provides the tools for an astute, caring physician to help you build the ship that will carry you toward a wellness lifestyle. This guidance can now be customized for you. Now, of course, the physician is going to suggest steps for improvement, longevity, or amelioration of present diseases; but it's really up to you to decide which course to take. Isn't that a unique technique? I'd hope not. The patient is at the helm of the ship, and it is by working together with a physician who understands those needs and goals that the best course can be charted.

Once that is done, it really does take a commitment on the part of the patient. In my practice, patients often keep a log. We follow their weight, blood pressure, mental status, goals reached, or any other defining parameters we are watching in this patient-kept log. It is only by writing it down that we are able to qualify and quantify how the patient is progressing in order to make necessary changes. Yeah, I'm really sorry, but you've *got* to do your part in this "getting a better you" thing as well.

During this entire wellness process, I use a mnemonic called BALANCE.

> (B) **The B is utilizing the bioidentical hormones that we've spoken about.** These help create the path that we want to take. If your goal is to lose weight, but your thyroid and testosterone are down and your estrogen is high, then weight loss is just not going to happen right now. We've got to put your testosterone, estrogen, and all the other hormones in alignment first.

> (A) **The A is for an appetite plan.** Now an appetite plan needs to be well-calculated and based on what your goals are. I hope you don't want to look like Twiggy because this program includes sanity. My goal for my patients is to bring their percentage of body fat into a range in which they have a maximally decreased risk of developing diabetes, coronary artery disease, stroke, or the like. That range is 15% to 25% body fat.

> (L) **The L is for longevity principles.** These include such entities as sleep, not smoking, decreased alcohol intake (only one 4-ounce drink per night), and other principles of wellness that are applicable to all of us. You may not want

to be a marathoner, so walking everyday will be the right path for you. Great—let's go for it! The next day, of course, we utilize another activity program. It's only by moving muscle that we can bring sugar into the muscles and out of fat cells. It's only by moving muscle that we can correct unbalanced hormones such as elevated estrogen levels and high insulin. We can increase testosterone and actually even increase thyroid function by simply moving muscle.

(A) **The next A is for an activity program.** It doesn't have to be a big deal. It can be morning semi-squats coming out of bed that is followed by a lunch of push-ups against the wall and nighttime over-the-shoulder exercises with two cans of tomato soup. It really doesn't matter. It just requires the movement of muscle. Want to take it to a higher level? Go for it—but remember for those of you who are in the go, go, go mode, your biggest threat is injury. Sanity is the key; and please remember that 15 to 30 minutes of daily resistance training or walking is sufficient.

(N) **The N is for nutraceuticals.** There is a set of effective nutraceuticals that can enhance your goals. For example, if you are diabetic and wish to improve your blood sugar, there are nutraceuticals such as selenium, alphalipoic acid, Omega-3, CoQ10, vanadium, and cinnamon that can be helpful sugar controllers. Of course, the key to controlling diabetes is decreasing sugar intake. If it's white, don't bite! Only eat a few fruits—yes, that's right, I said "few fruits." They're sugar! Bread, potatoes, corn—send them to those starving children in China who you were always told about by your parents. Keep your alcohol consumption low, and forget the diet soda and fruit or vegetable juice. Think of them as a Snickers bar: Enjoy them once a week, but not more frequently.

(C) **The C is for cognition.** Cognition is really the core in my
practice. We actually test patients for their neurotransmitter
levels. I utilize the levels that a patient has in terms of serotonin (calming), dopamine (cravings and multi-tasking),
GABA (enhancement of serotonin), and norepinephrine/
epinephrine (adrenalin) to help create the symphony of
balance. To enhance these neurotransmitters, we find what
their levels are and use natural essential amino acids and
neurotransmitter-specific supplements to raise their levels
when appropriate. For serotonin, we would certainly utilize
high B vitamins with vitamin C along with leucine, isoleucine, tryptophan, 5-HTP, tyrosine, and phenylalanine.
Now don't let the big words scare you. These are all simply
natural amino acids, but they are ones that we do not create within ourselves. We must ingest them. Stressors of all
kinds, of course, will deplete these amino acids rapidly, so
they must be replenished daily.

(E) **The E is for enjoyment.** The most important of all
elements for healthy living is the E—enjoyment. I can't
imagine having a goal or striving for any dream without
enjoyment in all forms being present. No, I'm not trying
to sound like a birthday card. I know we all have our ups
and downs, but keeping those ups and downs even is really
the essence of life. The big question is how do you do that?
That's probably the most common question that comes up
in my practice. I certainly don't have the guru answer, but I
can tell you what has worked for me. As you know, I have
had multiple medical problems in the past. I have had a
number of stressors in my life including ejecting from a
fighter jet and being shot down in Vietnam (twice). (Yeah,
I just wasn't that good of a pilot.) Surgical residencies,
family practice residences, preventive medicine, pain, and

bariatric fellowships all have taken their toll. So how do you stay happy? How do you get to enjoy life? Let's go a little deeper into that.

My path is very simple, but it requires a daily exercise. Just as if I wanted bigger biceps, I'd have to exercise them every day. I spoke before about my mnemonic GAGE. Remember? Gratitude, Acceptance, and Giving. All of those then equal Enjoyment. GAGE absolutely never fails to brighten my day. Add two compliments each day to my daughter and wife, and the enjoyment is guaranteed.

A few moments before my GAGE time is ideal time for me to treat myself to 5 or 10 minutes of meditation. Truthfully, if I spend longer than that, I feel as though I should shave my head. Now, what is meditation for me? Meditation is simply sitting in a comfortable chair (no, not pretzel-twisted in a yoga pose) and breathing. Let's see if you can remember what I do next. As I breathe in, I mentally say "accept." I then exhale, saying "aware" silently. It's a great way for me to accept the day and be aware of my connections to this day. This is a nice gift I also give myself in the middle of a hectic day.

You can also give yourself a couple of moments of meditation before sleep. No, you don't have to go into a Zen state. Simply feel your breath as it passes your nostrils. Maybe it'll only be five breaths. Maybe it'll only be a couple of minutes of silence. My daughter Kristy, a physician, taught me to verbalize three gratitudes at the end of the day. I now do this with my wife and my daughter Ellie—and yes, I share texts with Kristy. It acts like a massage!

Some final tidbits and reminders:

~ Floss. I used to hate it when my dentist said I needed to floss. Sorry, Dr. Witherby, but you were right. As I've said, flossing is really key to great dentition and good health. Remember how those lions died of gum disease and starvation? Sure, I'm all about saving the whales, but imagine what we could do by flossing the lions.

～ Practice your posture. For me, that's a toughie. I back up to a wall three or four times a day and try to straighten my posture. Good posture helps your breathing. It says to others, "I'm confident and in control." After a hard day of work, we come home with slumped shoulders. Why? Because we're carrying the weight of today. Practicing good posture during the day lets that weight fall off.

～ Covering your 6 o'clock. This is fighter-pilot lingo for watch your fanny! In flying combat, it was so easy to look ahead from your cockpit position. I had lots to look at and lots to look for. It is so easy to forget the position behind you. Was that a bogie swooping down on your tail that you just weren't watching for? It's no different with your healthcare. Let's watch out for our fannies in this maze of medical maelstrom.

～ Please remember that everyone, including your physician and your next door neighbor, is entitled to their own opinion. They are not, however, entitled to their own facts. Your physician may say that he THINKS you should be on a statin or a choles-terol-lowering medicine. Your response should be, "Thank you so much for your opinion, but what are the facts that indicate that it will not hurt me and that it will indeed prolong my life?" The response to your neighbor should be one of "thank you." Realize that what worked for your neighbor almost assuredly will not work for you.

～ Drugs and supplements kill. It's just a fact. Like I said before, the difference between a poison and a medicine is the amount or dose. Everything you put in your mouth needs to be scruti-nized, and you must know that what you are taking is for your benefit and not your harm.

～ In general, insurance companies are not your friend. They are a business, and their business is to hold on to their financial stakes. These stakes include your wallet. I'm sorry if I sound harsh, but the American system today has gone completely haywire. When an insurance company can dictate to me, a physician, how I treat a patient, something is dreadfully wrong. I'm sorry.

~ Always check your physician's bills and hospital bills. Computers and individuals make mistakes. There are no Phi Beta Kappas managing your invoice for medical procedures or care.

~ The best thing that you can take to a hospital if you are being admitted is a friend. You need someone to watch out and care for you in a system where there is often not enough time for the caring you need. Would you like to read but forgot your reading glasses? Nice to have a friend there to get them for you later. It's the little things that will need tending to.

~ The way you live is a choice. I'm really sorry that this is going to sound so corny, but after 68 years on this Earth, I've come up with a very important, indelible truth: You are what you think. Your day is your choice; your mood is your choice, and your beliefs are your choice. I guess I could go on further, but I'm sure you get my point. Choose today to give, and you will know enjoyment. Choose to smile when it's the hardest thing in the world for you to do, and you will smile inside as well. The job may fail; the bills will come; and disasters will happen. But the choice of how you deal with calamity can never be taken from you. Can't take another minute of the chaos that seems like an engulfing wave in your life? Give. Give of yourself, and give of your time—give of your heart. No, it won't make the bills go away or the cancer abate, but it will bring peace and warmth to your inner life. I guarantee it. Throw in a tablespoon of "This too shall pass," and your life will be enriched along with the lives of those you've touched.

My Big, Big Sorry

This book could be an encyclopedia, but we would both run out of time. I really am sorry that we can't cover everything. The good news is that you can always e-mail me with questions, and I will do my very best to answer them.

The important thing to remember is that you are working on you—not your spouse, but *you*. Remember that "doctor" means "teacher." Let's all become doctors. Teach your spouse, your children, and your friends. We need a national change to encourage and enhance wellness. Most importantly—no apology here—thank you for taking an interest in your health.

> *"Everyone wants to go to heaven, but nobody wants to die. In the end, you will die alone regardless of who was at your side. What will matter most will be how well you lived, how well you loved, how well you laughed, and how well you were able to let go."*—Me

The truth for healthy living:

> *"Any good that I can perform today, let me do it now. Please let me not defer or neglect it. For I shall not pass this way again."*—Anonymous

Appendix

Useful Websites

www.nih.gov

www.medscape.com

www.pubmed.com

www.worldhealth.net

www.glycemicindex.com

www.menshealth.com

www.womanshealthmag.com

www.functionalmedicine.org

www.worldhealth.net

www.a4m.com

Supplement Vendors/Labs

www.ihealthspan.com

www.syntrax.com

www.leanerliving.com

www.davincigourmet.com

www.lef.org (lab)

www.senesco.com (lab)

www.swansonvitamins.com

www.puritan.com

(For the validity of supplements and the companies selling them, please consult: www.consumerlab.com.)

Recommended Books on Nutrition

Fat Chance: Beating the Odds Against Sugar, Processed Food, Obesity, and Disease, Robert Lustig, M.D.

The Omnivore's Dilemma: A Natural History of Four Meals, Michael Pollan

Mindless Eating: Why We Eat More Than We Think, Brian Wansink, Ph.D.

Why We Get Fat: And What to Do About It, Gary Taubes

The New Atkins for a New You: The Ultimate Diet for Shedding Weight and Feeling Great, Eric Westman, M.D., Stephen Phinney, M.D., Jeff Volek, Ph.D.

The All-New Atkins Advantage, Stuart Trager, M.D. with Colette Heimowitz, M.Sc.

Atkins Diabetes Revolution, Robert Atkins, M.D., Mary Vernon, M.D., Jacqueline Eberstein, R.N.

The Paleo Solution: The Original Human Diet, Robb Wolf

The Paleo Diet Revised: Lose Weight and Get Healthy by Eating the Foods You Were Designed to Eat, Loren Cordain, Ph.D.

More Recommended Books

The UltraMind Solution: Fix Your Broken Brain by Healing Your Body First, Mark Hyman, M.D.

You Staying Young: The Owner's Manual for Extending Your Warranty, Michael Roizen, M.D., Mehmet Oz, M.D.

The Edge Effect: Achieve Total Health and Longevity with the Balanced Brain Advantage, Eric Braverman, M.D.

Younger You: Unlock the Hidden Power of Your Brain to Look and Feel 15 Years Younger, Eric Braverman, M.D.

Forever Ageless, Ron Rothenberg, M.D., Kathleen Becker, Kris Hart.

What You Must Know About Woman's Hormones, Pamela Smith, M.D.

What You Must Know About Vitamins, Minerals, Herbs & More: Choosing the Nutrients That Are Right for You, Pamela Smith, M.D.

Project GRACE, a Suncoast Hospice affiliate, helps families and the healthcare professionals who serve them with the advance care planning process. They provide educational programs, resources, and training to healthcare and legal professionals, clergy, community organizations and the general public on end-of-life healthcare decision-making.

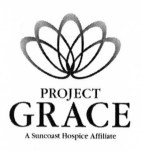

PROJECT
GRACE
A Suncoast Hospice Affiliate

Originally launched as an arm of the Florida Chapter of the American College of Cardiology (FCACC), Project GRACE was established through a partnership of physicians, care providers, ethicists and concerned citizens dedicated to changing the approach to end-of-life healthcare to be holistic, compassionate, respectful of human dignity and the individual's best interests and personal wishes.

Founders Dr. Lofty Basta and Dr. Henry D. McIntosh (both cardiologists) were passionately dedicated to empowering individuals and their loved ones to properly document their end-of-life medical decisions based on their own ethical, cultural and spiritual beliefs and values, affording them peace of mind, dignity and respect.

The best time to make decisions concerning your healthcare is while you are able to consider your wishes carefully and discuss them with your doctor, caregivers, family and loved ones. Advance Care Planning is a thoughtful process to plan for future healthcare choices, involving personal reflection and discussions about medical treatment preferences.

For additional information about advance care planning contact Project GRACE at 727–536–7364 or visit www.projectgrace.org.

Sample Advance Directive

Download the full-size form at: www.projectgrace.org

LIVING WILL &
APPOINTMENT OF HEALTHCARE SURROGATE

I, _____, want to choose how I will be treated by my physicians and other healthcare providers. If there comes a time when I am unable to communicate or make my own healthcare decisions because of illness or injury, I direct my physicians, my healthcare surrogate, and my family to honor this living will.

Part 1 – Appoint a Healthcare Surrogate

In the event I am unable to communicate or I am incapable of making decisions about receiving, withholding, or withdrawing medical procedures or other treatments, I designate my healthcare surrogate to make choices for me according to his/her understanding of my wishes and values.

My Appointed Healthcare Surrogate is:	
Name:	
Address:	
Phone:	Alt. Phone:

If my surrogate is unable or unwilling then my next choice (Alternate Surrogate) is:	
Name:	
Address:	
Phone:	Alt. Phone:

Part 2 – Indicate Your Wishes

I understand that this living will only becomes effective when I am no longer able to communicate or when I am not capable of making my healthcare decisions. When two physicians have determined that I have one of the following:

- a terminal or end-stage condition, and there is little or no chance of recovery
- a condition of permanent and irreversible unconsciousness, such as coma or vegetative state
- an irreversible and severe mental or physical illness that prevents me from communicating with others, recognizing my family and friends, or caring for myself in any way

then I want my doctors and others to provide comfort (palliative) care including relief of all physical pain, suffocation and mental anguish. If I develop one of the above conditions, my treatment choices are:

My Specific Choices if I have one of the above conditions	Yes I Want	No I Do Not Want
	Circle Yes or No	
Cardio-pulmonary resuscitation (CPR) if my heart or breathing stops	Yes	No
A breathing machine if I am unable to breathe on my own	Yes	No
Nutrition and fluids through tubes in my veins, nose or stomach	Yes	No
Kidney dialysis, a pacemaker or defibrillator, or other such machines	Yes	No
Surgery or admission to a hospital Intensive Care Unit	Yes	No
Medications that can prolong my dying, such as antibiotics	Yes	No
I want Hospice involved in my care at the earliest opportunity	Yes	No

Please copy both sides.   Page 1 of 2   © Project GRACE 2010

If a medical decision has to be made for me and my decision is not indicated above, I want my healthcare surrogate to make and communicate these decisions for me.

Other Information (optional):
Quality of life is important to me. These are the things that give my life quality:

_____

_____

_____

_____

_____

_____

_____

_____

Part 3 – Make It Legal

I fully understand the meaning of this declaration, I am emotionally and mentally competent to make this declaration, and have given this declaration careful consideration.

_____   _____   _____
            Signature   Date   Print Name

*Witness 1: _____   _____
                    Signature of witness 1   Print Name

Address: _____

*Witness 2: _____   _____
                    Signature of witness 2   Print Name

Address: _____

* Your healthcare surrogate(s) can not serve as a witness to this living will.
  At least one witness must be someone other than your spouse or a blood relative.

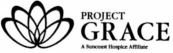

PROJECT
GRACE
A Suncoast Hospice Affiliate

5771 Roosevelt Blvd • Clearwater, FL 33760 • www.projectgrace.org • 727-536-7364

Example Diets

Sample 1200 Calorie Meal Planner

Qty	Measure	Description	Protein (gm)	Carbs (gm)	Fats (gm)	Calories
BREAKFAST						
2	Large	Egg, scrambled, hard-boiled, omelet	12.58	1.12	10.61	155.00
0.50	each	Grapefuit - pink or red	0.60	11.90	0.10	46.00
1	cup (8 fl oz)	Tea	0.00	0.71	0.00	2.37
		Totals:	13.18	13.73	10.71	203.37
AM SNACK						
2	1-in Cubes	Cheese, Cottage Cheese, String-Cheese, 2oz Nuts	14.00	1.00	14.00	180.00
		Totals:	14.00	1.00	14.00	180.00
LUNCH						
2	oz	Tuna, white, canned in water	16.44	0.00	1.00	70.00
0.50	each	Pita	1.40	7.80	0.35	37.50
0.5	cup	Spinach	0.29	0.50	0.04	3.50
3	slices	Tomato, sliced or diced or Green/ yellow/red peppers	0.53	2.35	0.12	10.80
		Totals:	18.66	10.65	1.51	121.80
PM SNACK						
0.50	each	Apple	0.15	10.50	0.25	40.50
0.50	cup	Yogurt or Hot Drink, Broth, Tea, Coffee	5.30	9.65	0.20	60.50
		Totals:	5.45	20.15	0.45	101.00
DINNER						
1	cup	Cauliflower	2.28	5.10	0.56	28.52
1	cup	Salad, green w/raw vegetables	1.73	4.44	0.10	22.00
1	TBSP	Oil & vinegar, WishBone, Lite Classic	0.00	2.00	2.00	20.00
6	oz	Salmon, broiled	37.62	0.00	21.00	348.00
		Totals:	41.63	11.54	23.66	418.52
EVENING SNACK						
1	Cup	Celery Sticks	2.00	5.00	0.20	20.00
2	1-in Cubes	Cheese, Cottage Cheese, String-Cheese, 2oz Nuts	14.00	1.00	14.00	180.00
		Totals:	16.00	6.00	14.20	200.00
		Actual Totals	108.92	63.07	64.53	1224.69

Sample 1500 Calorie Meal Planner

Qty	Measure	Description	Protein (gm)	Carbs (gm)	Fats (gm)	Calories
BREAKFAST						
0.5	cup	Blueberries	0.27	5.25	0.12	20.66
2	1-in Cubes	Cheese, Cottage Cheese, String-Cheese, 2oz Nuts	14.00	1.00	14.00	180.00
		Totals:	14.27	6.25	14.12	200.66
AM SNACK						
1	scoop	Whey or Egg Protein Shake	23.00	3.00	2.00	120.00
		Totals:	23.00	3.00	2.00	120.00
LUNCH						
2	oz	Tuna, white, canned in water	16.44	0.00	1.00	70.00
1	TBSP	Pickle relish or olive spread	0.03	1.33	0.03	5.00
0.5	cup	Spinach	0.29	0.50	0.04	3.50
3	slices	Tomato, sliced or diced or Green/ yellow/red peppers	0.53	2.35	0.12	10.80
		Totals:	17.29	4.18	1.19	89.30
PM SNACK						
1	scoop	Whey or Egg Protein Shake	23.00	3.00	2.00	120.00
1.00	each	Apple	0.30	21.00	0.50	81.00
		Totals:	23.30	24.00	2.50	201.00
DINNER						
2	TBSP	BBQ Sauce - Healthy Choice	0.06	11.40	0.04	50.00
1	TBSP	Olive Oil	0.00	0.00	14.00	130.00
2	3-oz	Pork tenderloin, roasted	47.84	0.00	8.18	278.80
1	small	Salad, garden w/tomato and onion	1.30	9.50	0.40	49.00
1	cup	Green Beans	2.00	8.00	0.47	41.40
		Totals:	51.20	28.90	23.09	549.20
EVENING SNACK						
2	1-in Cubes	Cheese, Cottage Cheese, String-Cheese, 2oz Nuts	14.00	1.00	14.00	180.00
1	cup	Jello w/ Cool Whip	0.00	19.00	1.00	88.00
		Totals:	14.00	20.00	15.00	268.00
		Actual Totals	143.06	86.33	57.90	1428.16

Sample 1800 Calorie Meal Planner

Qty	Measure	Description	Protein (gm)	Carbs (gm)	Fats (gm)	Calories
BREAKFAST						
2	Slices	Bacon	3.00	0.00	4.00	46.98
2	1-in Cubes	Cheese, Cottage Cheese, String-Cheese, 2oz Nuts	14.00	1.00	14.00	180.00
2	Large	Egg, scrambled, hard-boiled, omelet	12.58	1.12	10.61	155.00
1	cup (8 fl oz)	Tea	0.00	0.71	0.00	2.37
		Totals:	29.58	2.83	28.61	384.35
AM SNACK						
1	scoop	Whey or Egg Protein Shake	23.00	3.00	2.00	120.00
0.5	cup	Strawberries	0.50	4.50	0.00	30.00
		Totals:	23.50	7.50	2.00	150.00
LUNCH						
2	oz	Tuna, white, canned in water	16.44	0.00	1.00	70.00
0.50	each	Pita, wheat	1.40	7.80	0.35	37.50
0.5	cup	Spinach	0.29	0.50	0.04	3.50
0.50	cup	Tomato, sliced or diced	0.38	2.09	0.15	9.50
		Totals:	18.51	10.39	1.54	120.50
PM SNACK						
0.25	each	Apple	0.08	5.25	0.13	20.25
2	TBSP	Peanut Butter, all natural, creamy	8.00	6.00	16.00	210.00
		Totals:	8.08	11.25	16.13	230.25
DINNER						
1	cup	Cauliflower	2.28	5.10	0.56	28.52
1	cup	Salad, green w/raw vegetables	1.73	4.44	0.10	22.00
2	TBSP	Oil & vinegar, WishBone, Lite Classic	0.00	4.00	4.00	40.00
6	oz	Salmon, wild, broiled	37.62	0.00	21.00	348.00
1	Large	Deviled Egg	6.00	1.00	16.00	178.00
		Totals:	47.63	14.54	41.66	616.52
EVENING SNACK						
1	scoop	Whey or Egg Protein Shake	23.00	3.00	2.00	120.00
1	slice	Angel Food Cake w/Sugar Free Cool Whip	0.00	38.00	1.00	150.00
		Totals:	23.00	41.00	3.00	270.00
		Actual Totals	150.30	87.51	92.94	1771.62

Acknowledgements

Adam, Becca, Matt, William, Rusty, Bob, Julian, George, Eric, Mort, Mary, Beth, Silvia, Rhonda, Rose, Jupe, Frank, Ellen, Dan, Brent, Reesa, Roger, Martin, Jaimie, Chip, Debbie, Antonio, Tom Jr., Hank, Ashton, John, Darrell, Nancy, Kim, Skye, Danny, Libby, Bill, Ron, Sue, India, Cathy, Jack, and ... You!